TANTRIC SEX
Guide for Couples

Explore the Path of Sacred Sex to Reach the Ultimate Pleasure.
Spice Up Your Sex Life Through Meditation, Breathing, and
Illustrated Tantra Sex Positions

SAMANTHA MANDALA

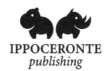

IPPOCERONTE
publishing

Cover designed by thiwwy design (@thiwwy) and Anne-marie Ridderhof from Pixabay, Photo by Chris Yang (@chrisyangchrisfilm) on Unsplash. Book Formatting designed by macrovector / Freepik, rawpixel.com / Freepik, and thiwwy design.

CONTENTS

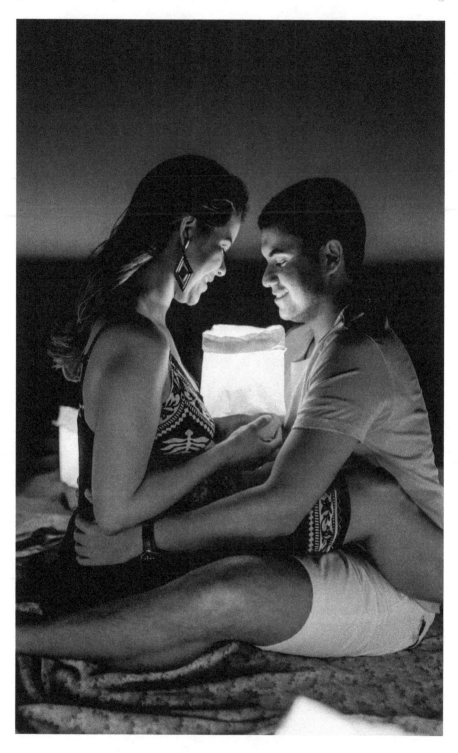

Introduction

We learn about sex in school and build it in our imagination through stories, movies, novels, and commercials. But the intercourse showed by the media is often an exaggeration: the whole circumstances are often extreme but romantic, and the act of sex itself is like a take-breath-away experience imagined with firecrackers and flashes.

This visualization of sex may cause pressure in ordinary life, and real people may want to perform like the characters they see in those movies. This sort of portrayal has set in individuals' psyches significantly elevated requirements that are hard to accomplish in reality, particularly from young couples who need insight.

When the experience isn't just about as high as envisioned, individuals may feel disappointed and lose self-assurance. Likewise, they may believe that the entire relationship has lost its enthusiasm and is near the precarious edge of self-destructing.

Simultaneously, sex sometimes is a level battleground. We might be searching for sexual intimacy at the core of our being, yet in addition, we take incredible consideration to evade it. Maybe we need to be contacted with our entire heart yet dread our shortcomings. We may take longer to recover lost energy yet have failed to remember how to light the fire.

From what I can see, there is a significant misreading of sex inside the western culture because the sexual education given to us since our best age is limited to only physical and biological activity. Sex could be much more than an instinct that pushes creatures to procreate, and it's also much more than an activity for "having a great time." Sex can be an instrument to explore our body and our way to pleasure, and it's also the best venture to connect with our partner.

In some east cultures, lovemaking is a ritual that deals not only with the physical world but also with the spiritual one. And this is what we call Tantra.

Tantra is not the mere act of sex made to please ourselves and our partner. Instead, it's a whole journey that carries humans close to the divinities using the "dance" of our bodies.

Whatever you are looking for a spiritual journey or just for suggestions to get the best experience from the act of love, Tantra can help you explore yourself and to learn more about pleasure and discover what you like. Learning about Tantra is also the best way to improve the relationship between couples since this discipline teaches the path to knowledge through the connection with a partner.

The way of thinking of Tantra shows us how to recuperate our sexual intimacy. Also, with this ancient practice, we can discover new sensual delights and change simple snapshots of sexual pleasure into the existence of sexual ecstasy.

When everyday stress, fears, and interruptions compromise relationships, Tantra practice shows us how to open our hearts, get in touch with our emotions and sexuality.

With everything on the planet today being rushed, hurried,

and loaded with pressure, we don't invest sufficient energy appreciating the pleasure. Easy-going sex and quick ones have supplanted intimacy and love, and it appears that nobody has "the time" any longer to live sex how it was intended to.

Sex is not only a physical act; it is two souls meeting up to make a sexual encounter that rises above the actual limits. Tantric sex is an action where couples participate in different sexually and sincerely fulfilling encounters to help blend their spirits.

The tantric sex approach takes things gradually, appreciating each experience and getting a charge out of it. It's not tied in with achieving an orgasm, yet it teaches to enjoying the intimacy you share with your accomplice. Sex shouldn't be an exhibition that simply makes a cursory effort. Where's the association, the love, the intimacy, and the uncommon bond that is possibly divided among lovers when it doesn't convert into your sex life? Lovemaking is far beyond the actual demonstration of sex; it is about creating a bond with your partner.

I know there are many books regarding this matter, and I would like to thank you for your trust in choosing this one! I decided to write this book to share my knowledge about this fascinating topic that opened my mind to new experiences. Like many, I had an ordinary life, spending my life between job, family, and friends. Eventually, I started to lose enthusiasm; even sex couldn't cheer me up. It was when sharing these feelings with one of my friends that he introduced me to Tantra. In the beginning, it was just a game, but I soon realized that our encounters didn't end in bed, but they were bringing benefits into my everyday life. To be specific, my life wasn't changing; I was the one that was seeing things differently because I slowly started to open myself to this world.

Sometimes we need a spark to change our life. Tantra was my spark. It helped me light my everyday routine, find meaning in my existence, and enjoy every pleasure fully.

This book takes the reader on a steady restorative excursion, clarifying the interconnectivity of the activities of your brain, soul, body, climate, and feelings to investigate with your accomplice. Whenever utilized effectively, it can get a special proclivity and put some extra spice in your relationship. Similar to yoga, it plans to locate the correct equilibrium and importance throughout everyday life.

~ CHAPTER 1 ~
Tantra, Meaning and Origins

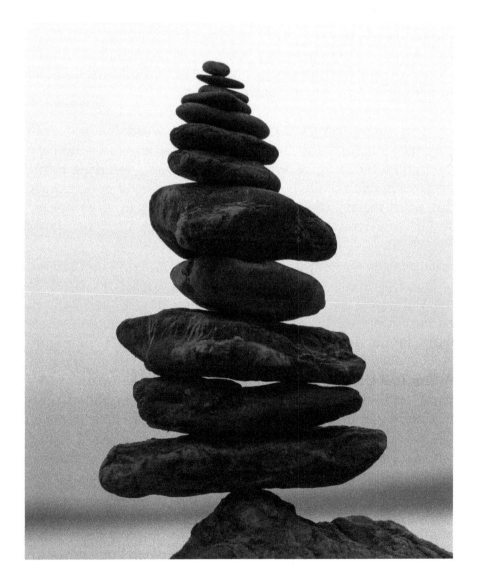

1.1 WHAT IS TANTRA?

Tantra is a way of thinking that arose in India around the 6th century; it has been connected to progressive influxes of progressive ideas, from its initial change of Hinduism and Buddhism to the Indian battle for autonomy and the ascent of 1960s nonconformity.

The Sanskrit word 'Tantra' comes from the verbal root *tan*, signifying 'to weave,' or 'form,' like the warping of threads on a loom. It refers to sacred texts, which we can find in both Hinduism and Buddhist religions. The same Buddhist texts are sometimes referred to as Tantra or sutra.

Each of those Indian texts applies the word 'Tantra' with various contextual and interpretations. In some cases, it keeps its original meaning of 'wave,' 'warp,' 'loom,' referring to the deep connection of the body and the spirit. On other occasions, this word means 'discipline,' 'rituals and practices,' 'essence,' and in some cases even 'doctrine' and 'science.'

Because of so many applications, Tantra has always had a broad range of meanings and teachings. Therefore, it is not possible to think of Tantra as a single practice, philosophy, or path without encountering people who disagree with you. Nonetheless, the word 'tantra' does refer to something coherent and meaningful.

Asana, mantra, pranayama, reflection, and rituals are the crucial parts of Tantra. These components blended in the various schools where each school varies from the others since it moves the accentuation on some element or another. As a result, tantrism significantly influenced many religions, including Shavis, Buddhism, Vaishnavism, and Jainism.

Some people see Tantra as a kind of "Yoga for sex," which, in my opinion, it would be a superficial and incomplete description by far. Regardless, the part of sex in this discipline shows up only occasionally in the sacred texts.

Other people would rather see it as a religion, which still won't be correct, even if the Tantric symbology and practices have emerged throughout history in many religions and cultures. Tantra may depend on mystical ideas, but it leads to an elevation of the spirit only through the exploration of the human body.

So, forgive me if my definition of Tantra doesn't cover all the meanings acquired in centuries through religious practice and cultural influence over different territories. Probably a whole book won't be enough to cover the meaning of this discipline in all its parts, but for sure, you'll get a better understanding going through this book. For now, consider Tantra as an experience that allows you to explore yourself with your body. You can see it as a journey that will help you to find pleasure in your everyday life.

Thinking about Buddhism, I can even say that, if done correctly, Tantra may even help you to reach the illumination. For example, one of the primary objectives of Buddhism is to overcome desire because it leads to a path of frustration and despair since humans can't be fully satisfied.

The ideal approach to accomplish this is to experience the passion and train it so we would be able to control it. Therefore, whenever utilized accurately, Tantra could show individuals the pathway to accomplish enlightenment.

In some cultures, people believe that some monks or gurus managed to achieve empowerment from this discipline. Like a healthy body and long life, without mentioning a profound elevation of the spirit.

Without a doubt, the tantric methodology assists with mitigating the pressure of the couple. Furthermore, it will give the correct guidance to forget about the "execution tension" and provide an alternative practice where you can discover your pleasure alongside your partner.

1.2 TANTRA TEXTS

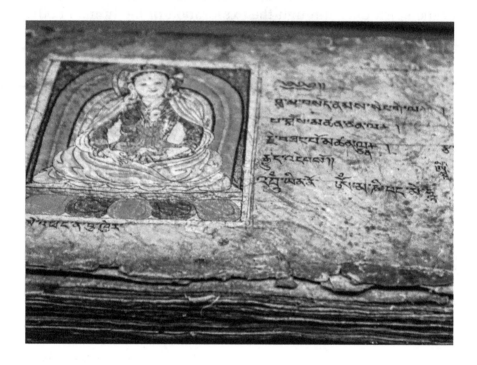

Two primary ancient texts inspired Indian philosophy: Vedas and Tantras. Composed in Sanskrit, the texts constitute the oldest layer of Sanskrit literature and the oldest scriptures of Hinduism. There is still a considerable debate on which one came first, but it is clear that they were born a long time before their transcription as they were initially passed orally.

Even if those two sacred texts aim to reach illumination, they have some disagreement on the approach to apply for the enlightenment. Still, the differences between the two are so minor that sometimes people confuse one with the other.

To see the differences between the two, we should get deep into the details. Still, we can summarize by saying that Tantra exalts individual power and recommended practice, while Vedas gives more authority to collective energy based on rituals in groups. Many people think that the present day of spiritual practices in India is based on Vedas. But in reality, a majority of the rituals and practices are based on Tantra and partly on Vedas.

There are two categories of these sacred texts: Agama and Nigama. Vedas literature is referred to as Nigama and is understood as the highest truth, describing the origin of creation itself. Agamic texts were written much later than Vedas, and the meaning of Agama is "that which has come." The Agamas neither accept nor reject the Vedas, but they use the knowledge revealed in Nigama for appropriate practices.

There are three types of Agamas:

1. Vaishnava Agamas – worship and regard Vishnu as the supreme
2. Shaiva Agamas – worship and regard Shiva as the supreme
3. Shakta Agamas – worship and regard Divine Mother (Shakti) as the supreme

Those texts are the transposition of divine dialogues as the gods themselves wrote them. In particular, the divines Shiva and Shakti or their emanations talking in-person in the sutras, as a conversation between husband and wife where one is asking questions and the other is teaching, as a relationship between student and teacher.

Technically, talking about tantras, we refer to the Shakta Agamas, where the Goddess Shakti has the teacher's role and reveals the knowledge of the creation to the God Shiva.

Tantric texts are written in aphorisms to express complex and ideological concepts that are subjected to different interpretations. This literature has mostly more than one reading and can be experienced at varying levels of intuition. Thus, the same text may be confusing or illuminating, depending on the reader's level of experience.

Today we can count more than 500 existing Tantras, but many of them have not been translated from Sanskrit. We believe that initially, there were more than 14000 volumes and that most of them have been lost over time.

Even if each text is open to different interpretations, it cannot be said that the tantric texts contradict each other; they just give importance to various aspects than others.

1.3 FROM THE ORIGIN TO TODAY

There have been various attempts to determine the origin of Tantra. According to some historians, the first appearance of the tantric practice in the first sacred text is dated around 600 CE. However, some indications show that Tantra may have started its journey from the Bronze Age, around 2000 BC. In this period, the civilization populating the Indus Valley Region was the Harappan from Harappa, the first urban center discovered by archeologists in this territory. This culture was probably the first to build at least one bathroom in their homes, something unheard of for the other civilizations in the same era. They also made a swimming pool in the heart of their capital Mohenjo-Daro, instead of using it as a center for governance and commerce.

Another peculiarity of this civilization is the privileged role that women kept in both society and religion. Statues and items picturing a female figure with open arms and legs spread apart were found in many sanctuaries and buildings. These representations are showing the woman as the mother goddess offering herself to adoration.

It is believed that the woman was the center of the Tantra culture, and for this reason, ladies are allowed to teach the tantra dogma. At the same time, in other religions, like Hinduism, female teachers were forbidden.

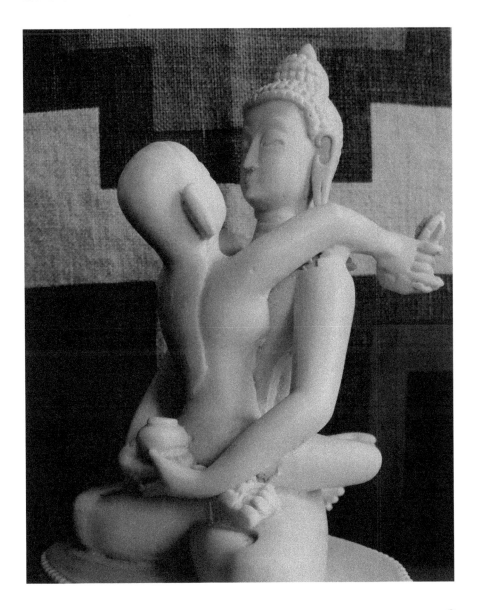

Talking about Tantra, there are two different paths that its practitioners describe: *Dakshinachara* and *Vamachara*.

Dakshinachara is translated as Right-Hand Path and is also known as *white Tantra*. It consists of the traditional practices where enlightenment is reached through asceticism and meditation. White Tantra is an esoteric female-focused tradition, which emphasizes meditation over other practices. The goal of the right path is not to get closer to a deity or achieve liberation from life or death; instead, practitioners focus on their individual journey by uncovering and purifying the mind. White tantric practitioners typically work within four categories: Wisdom Practice, Magical Practice, Mental Practice, and Emotional Practice. Hinduism, Tibetan Buddhism, Kundalini, and Kriya yoga are right-handed paths, all of which follow the traditional tantric practices described.

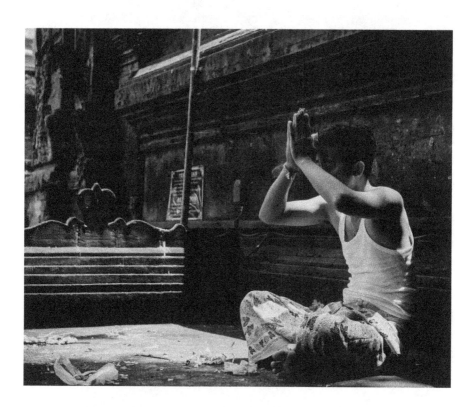

Vamachara is instead the Left-Hand Path, also known as *red Tantra*, and it includes ritual practices in contrast with the white Tantra. Vamachara is attached to materiality and sexual instincts, and this path ritual sex, alcohol, and other intoxications are allowed. It is based on the belief that sexuality can be used in a spiritual and ritualistic way to achieve union with the Divine. Devotees of red Tantra believe that this union can be achieved with any human of any gender. Sexual energy is an element shared with boths the paths but used for different purposes. The final goal of red tantra is to create a profound connection with the partner, while the white path is mostly a solitary journey. Both the paths can bring the *Moksha* (literally 'liberation' or 'nirvana'), but the Vamachara is mainly considered the fastest path.

The alleged "right hand" and "left hand" ways are unmistakably recognized. In the "right hand" path, the male and female divinities becoming one unity is considered an analogy at an energy level. In contrast, the "left hand" methods apply this allegoric image to the physical world.

Subsequently begins *maithuna* - the mysterious custom of love - which isn't a focal practice, although Tantra is today usually connected to it. On the opposite, *maithuna* is viewed as one of the most important and last stages that the yogi should confront because lone genuine yogis can stand to rehearse it as a contemplation method.

1.4 What is Neotantra?

The terminology 'Tantra' arrived in the West in conjunction with the sexual liberation of the 60s and 70s, and women's emancipation helped this teaching spread in America.

Neotantra is a recent and western form of Tantra that has been around for over 150 years. It does take inspiration from Hindu and

Buddhist ideas, but instead of focusing on reaching enlightenment, it pays attention primarily to sex and having a better orgasm. Neotantra is definitely a path inspired by Tantra, even if the two practices have different bases. The strong contrasts between them are: Neotantra depends on present-day books rather than old sacred writings and doesn't need a master for inception. In traditional Indian and Tibetan Tantra, a pioneer (alluded to as a *guru parampara*) is proclaimed as having the most extreme need for spiritual movement. Neotantrics fervently debate this, enticing the idea that anybody anxious to communicate sexually may start on their tantric way.

In contemporary occasions, the most well-known misconception is the qualification among Tantra and tantric sex. Tantra's derivation signifies 'the weaving and development of energy,' yet Tantra itself doesn't include sex by any means as opposed to mainstream thinking. Instead, it's teaching about the union of the manly and ladylike energy that can be accomplished through meditation and breathing procedures.

Its inceptions have been followed in the conventional writings of Hinduism, Buddhism, and other Asian convictions where sexual investigation has frequently been illegal, especially for ladies.

Tantric sex is the point at which these teachings are applied in the room. The matter becomes to develop a more private association among accomplices and a woven association with the Divine. The training isn't 'objective orientated,' yet somewhat a type of love looking to keep its members present all through. While tantric ecstasy and accomplishing the big O may end up happening simultaneously, they are unquestionably not a similar accomplishment.

When most people, especially in Western countries, talk about Tantra these days, they are actually talking about Neotantra. It is likewise intriguing to note that from the mid-late 20th century, as India was fighting for autonomy and finding new support over their public personality, Neotantra turned into a word habitually used to give India attention and merit, spread especially among the Western crowds.

While in 2018, Tantra got inseparable from "spiritual sex" and "holy sexuality," these semantics are dug in undeniably more unpredictable verifiable convictions. Similarly, as with most components of history notwithstanding, mindfulness and appreciation are vital.

Neaotranta is an adapted version of Tantra for the Occidentals, but it does help to spread some of the Eastern values into the Western world.

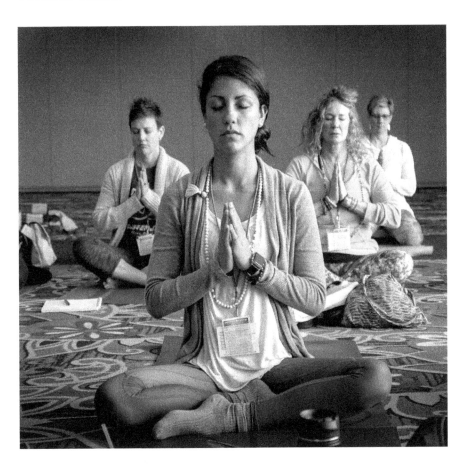

~ CHAPTER 2 ~

Tantra and Spirituality

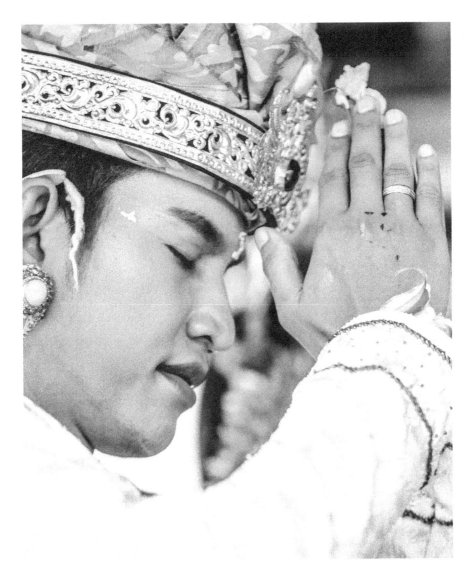

2.1 Tantra and the Way of Liberation

Tantra is a spiritual way and a lifestyle. It's an individual act of freedom. The act of Tantra frees you up to a spiritual encounter and to understanding the human body and natural life as tangible signs of divine energy. Sexual energy can be an incredible way to spiritual advancement. Life can be incorporated and celebrated on the way to illumination. The Tantric conviction that encountering sexual fervor is a sample of cosmic energy is a significant and progressive idea, as pertinent today as before. Tantra is the method of freedom that opens up to the genuine articulation of oneself.

The Guhyasamaja Tantra expresses that: "nobody can accomplish freedom on the off chance that he participates in troublesome and torturing practices; freedom is reachable through the cognizant satisfaction, everything being equal."

Tantra is a guide that teaches how to find the fulfillment and happiness that comes from being in harmony with your true nature. A path based on three principles:

- Knowledge: The more we know, the better equipped we are.
- Renunciation: The less clinging, the less suffering.
- Concentration: Hold it tight, like a fist. The result of this is our mental and physical health.

Tantra is the same path that was taught by all the Enlightened Masters who have ever pointed the way to liberation, from the time of Gautama Buddha to Jesus Christ, to Mohammed. What has been called "Tantric Yoga" is not a thing in itself, but essentially it is the Buddhist path in its esoteric (Vajrayana) form. The Vajrayana Buddhism of Tibet may restate the Mahayana teachings for those ready for more advanced work on this spiritual path.

Tantra is an ancient yogic practice that helps one achieve a deep meditative consciousness and personal transformation. It can also be used to transform relationships, both with oneself and with a partner.

Tantric practices are based on the fundamental understanding that sexuality is much more than the act of intercourse or genital stimulation. Instead, it is an exchange of energy between two people on all levels: spiritual, emotional, intellectual, and physical. Furthermore, Tantra teaches that this energy can be transmitted through touch to create ecstatic feelings of pleasure for both partners.

Tantra can revitalize even the most "tired" relationships and add new life to sexual expression when practiced regularly. Tantra can also overcome performance anxiety in new or established relationships by focusing on the physical sensations.

Tantric practices can be incorporated into any relationship – married, single, straight or gay. However, the benefits of practicing Tantra are most profound in long-term committed relationships because these are the relationships that have time to evolve and sustain themselves on all levels.

The effects of Tantra are most powerful if both partners practice. However, if one of the partners is not open to practicing Tantra, the benefits can still be significant for the other, especially for women.

2.2 THE SEVEN CHAKRAS

"When your chakras are balanced, you can experience clarity, access power, and feel more joyful, fearless, and free"
Jesse Lucier (2015).

If you dive into Tantra or any spiritual practice coming from the East, you'll face how mind and body are balanced together through masses of energy called chakras.

A chakra is a spinning wheel of energy. When it's spinning fast and in balance with other chakras, you're living in the present moment. But when your chakras get out of whack, life can start to feel constrained and heavy.

Those energy centers interact with the human body by numerous fibers, channels, and energy pathways. They're like the veins of a leaf: every leaf has many veins, but together they all stem from the same trunk. The power lies in how everything works together as a system.

The chakras are like the leaves of a tree: they radiate outward from the same source (the trunk). The power comes from how everything is interconnected and works together as a system. If one of your chakras is out of balance, then it will affect everything else in your life.

There are seven main chakras in the human body that all have their specific purposes and energies. These chakras are located on the back, from base to head. They're also associated with the human body's major organs, and each one of them has a specific color:

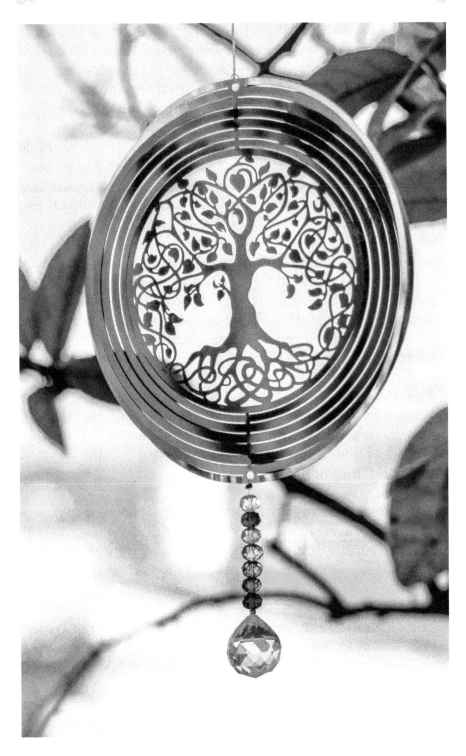

1. **Root Chakra – Muladhara (red):** The root chakra is located at the base of your spine, around the tailbone area. This chakra deals with feelings of intimacy, sex drive, security, self-esteem, and safety in relationships. It's the foundation center of the human body, giving stability and confidence.

2. **Sacral Chakra – Swadhisthana (orange):** This chakra is placed near the tailbone in your lower abdomen (below your belly button). The sacral chakra controls sexual pleasure and creativity as well as forming healthy connections with others. It also helps you find joy in everyday life.

3. **Solar Plexus Chakra – Manipura (yellow):** The solar plexus chakra can be found in the upper abdomen, just below your rib cage. This chakra deals with self-confidence, self-esteem, personal power, and the ability to stand up for oneself. It also helps you find the center when you're confused or feel off balance.

4. **The Heart Chakra – Anahata (green):** The heart chakra belongs in the center of your chest behind your breast bone. This chakra deals with love and compassion, as well as emotional intelligence. It also controls what you put out into the world: love or hate.

5. **The Throat Chakra – Vishuddha (blue):** The throat chakra is located in the middle of your throat. It deals with how you express yourself, from body language to how you speak. Learning to control this chakra will help you become a more expressive communicator.

6. **The Third Eye Chakra – Ajna (indigo):** This chakra is located between your eyes, and it deals with intuition, psychic abilities, and spiritual enlightenment. It's also responsible for making critical decisions, as well as self-control and balancing your thoughts and emotions.

7. **The Crown Chakra – Sahasrara (violet):** The crown chakra is placed near the top of your head. This chakra deals with spirituality, self-love, and letting go of the ego. It allows you to be connected to the cosmos and feel at peace within yourself.

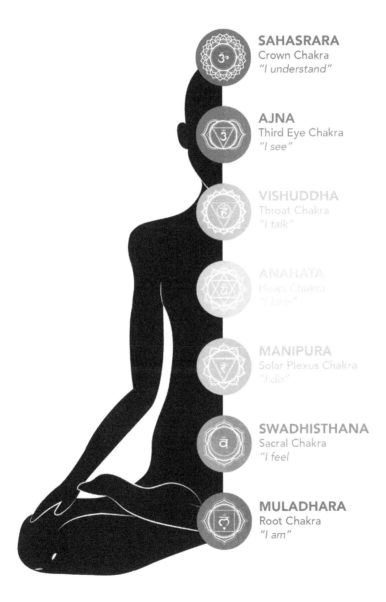

SAHASRARA
Crown Chakra
"I understand"

AJNA
Third Eye Chakra
"I see"

VISHUDDHA
Throat Chakra
"I talk"

ANAHATA
Heart Chakra
"I love"

MANIPURA
Solar Plexus Chakra
"I do"

SWADHISTHANA
Sacral Chakra
"I feel

MULADHARA
Root Chakra
"I am"

~ CHAPTER 3 ~
Complete Yourself With Your partner

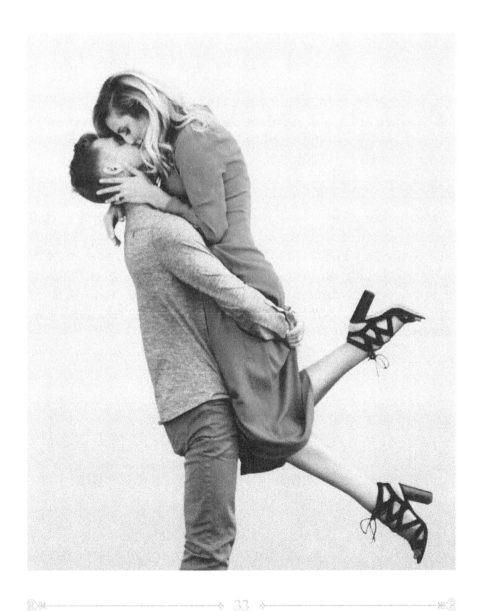

3.1 SEX AS SACRED ENERGY

In numerous, western and eastern cultures, sex is considered one of the most potent sacred energies, second to none. The thought that bound together these ancient cultures was that everything in the universe comes from sexual energy.

In India, Tibet, and China, this assembled vision arrives at its apogee: the divinities are addressed together and frequently in the situation of the caring demonstration. In Tantra, as in the other spiritual ways, the sexual dimension takes different shapes. Sometimes a couple of gods is represented lying down, like resting, sometimes they are in a sitting position, and in other times they are standing. These sacred icons represent the link between the earthly world and the spiritual and transformational world.

The sexual relationship, which is at the beginning of the entire existence, clarifies how every new life comes from a sexual demonstration. The beat and mood of love are present in each part of life as a cycle, vibration, or pulse. It is the alteration of the seasons and the movements of the planets; it is the beat of the heart and breath. Therefore, all presence is a nonstop innovative demonstration that emerges from the relentless love relationship of cognizance and energy.

3.2 SHIVA AND SHAKTI

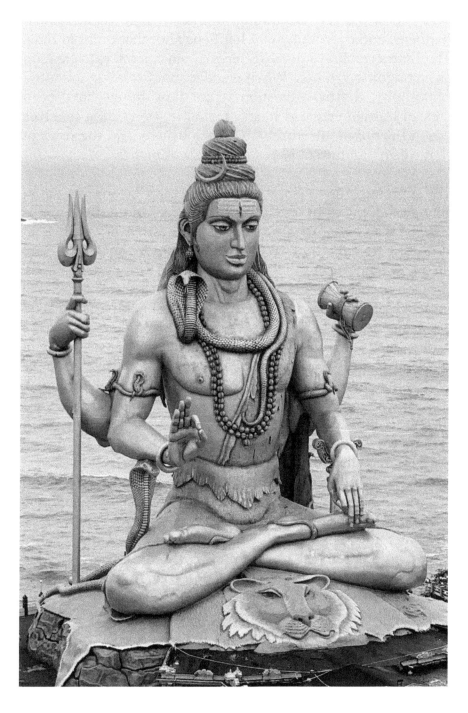

Every culture and religion has its own creation story; most of the ones that I'm familiar with usually narrate an event that occurred at the very beginning of time. This is when creation happens, and everything else happens after that point in time. The Tantra creation story is different; in fact, it refers to creation as an ongoing process. When we talk about creation in tantric philosophy, the first question is not how things have been created but who created them. In Tantra, everything revolves around *Brahman*, the supreme consciousness, and the concept that we are not the subject of our life; Brahman is.

The supreme consciousness is dreaming our existence the entire time and doing with us whatever it desires to do. Brahman is not just the God of the universe, but it is also every particle in it. Tantric religion thinks that all the entities in the universe are all expressions of Brahma. Also, according to Tantra, Brahman is made of two fundamental principles, *Shiva* and *Shakti*. Shiva is also called *Purusa* (consciousness), while Shakti can be called *Prakrti* (energy). Philosophically doesn't mean that God can be broken into two parts. It just means that there are two sides of the same God. We can say that Purusa is the cognitive principle of Brahman while Prakrti is the operative principle of Brahman.

Trying to explain this in just a few words is not simple, but I will give it a try. According to Tantra, God is always observing everything, but at the same time, God is being everything and is doing everything. When God is watching, then Brahman is in the role of Shiva (Purusa), and when is he is doing something, then he is in the role of Shakti (Prakrti). We can see Purusa as something that is static and never changes, while Prakrti is in constant change, and it multiplies. Prakrti acts as a bind for Purusa; It puts Purusa in certain constraints according to Purusa's will. We can say that Shakti (Prakrti) allows Shiva (Purusa) to express itself according to the three Gunas (binding principles): Sattvaguna, Rajoguna, and Tamoguna.

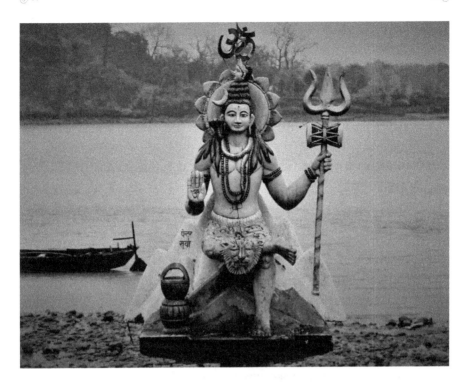

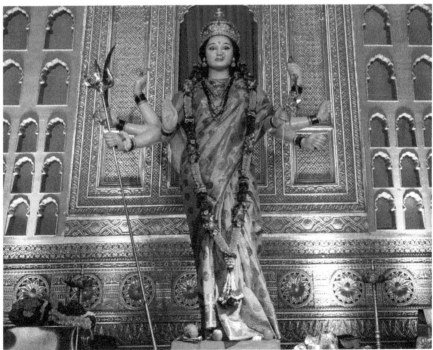

These are the three expressions of Brahman and the qualities you might find in every aspect of the universe.

- **Sattvaguna** means sentient, and it expresses the feeling of "I exist." This is how Shiva becomes aware of itself.
- **Rajoguna** means mutative, and it expresses the feeling of "I do."
- **Tamagun** means static, and it expresses the feeling of "I've done."

These three expressions, "I exist," "I do," and "I've done," are mental expressions, and we can infer that out of consciousness, it comes "mind."

So, if consciousness came first and it lately obtained the mind, what will naturally come next? According to Tantra, the matter was created next. Everything we can see, everything that is part of the universe, was made after consciousness acquired mind.

We can draw a parallel here with the big bang theory. According to this theory, the universe was generated from a single location and is, since then, in constant expansion. According to the Tantra, consciousness is in continuous expansion, obtaining a mind and later turning into the matter.

The big bang theory also says that time and space were the first things to exists before the matter was created, while in Tantra, we say that consciousness and mind came before matter.

These are just some similarities between the big bang theory and tantra, but let's now leave behind the theory of tantric creation to see the relation between Shiva and Shakti in more detail.

According to *Shaivism*, one of the branches of yogic philosophy, we can see Shiva as divine masculine energy while Shakti is considered divine feminine energy. Since Shiva and Shakti are an integral part of Brahman, they are also alive in every man and woman. We can say that everyone has divine masculine traits (Shiva) and divine feminine traits (Shakti); accessing them is not easy, but it can be an enlightening and surprising experience. Shiva is forever in union with Shakti, his divinely feminine consort; the nature of Shiva's energy is steadfast, stable, peaceful, strong, and totally unmoved with complete presence. It represents the state of being unaffected by pain or suffering brought on by the external world.

All the things of creation are generated through the feminine aspect of Shakti; her energy is dance, movement, power, energy, and the freedom to change. We can say that Shiva is a pure being in its stillness while Shakti is pure becoming in all her flow and creativity and her endless opening to possibility. Shakti is fluid, flowing, and powerfully flexible; her energy can be wildly sensual, raw, and expressive.

One of the main differences between their energies is that Shiva's energy is formless, while Shakti's energy can be seen in all things. These two energies are equal and opposite forces; we can't have one without the other, but we will see this concept in more detail in the following chapters.

3.3 YIN AND YANG - UNDERSTANDING THE OPPOSITES

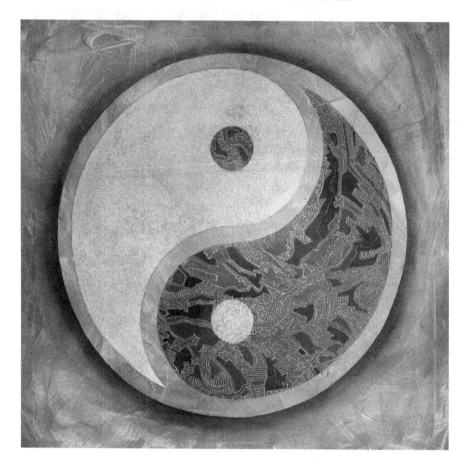

Since the fusion of Shiva and Shakti is the origin of the creation itself, these two entities are sometimes represented together as two halves of the same body, called *Ardhanarishvara*. This image is the synthesis of masculine and feminine energies of everything in the universe. It illustrates how the two forces are inseparable from each other but yet in the perfect balance. This tantric, unitary and transformative vision expanded from India to Tibet and China, where it assumes the image of Tao wherein the two polar powers Yin and Yang in balance. The Taoists' and tantric paths have some similarities: they accept mindfulness as the core of everything. They both recognize the equilibrium of female and male in each element and creature in the universe.

As indicated by the essential tantric standards, sex consolidates female energy and male energy and makes their union a blast, leading the two sides to rise. Reaching the highest pleasure is the final goal. Yet, there are additional halfway objectives, for example, freeing oneself up to love, improving collaboration with the partner, personally feeling the other as though they are one and the other.

To apply what is necessary to allow the couple to open to the Infinite (or possibly part of it), it is fundamental that the two sections are "spellbound," one of Yang (male) energy and the other of Yin (female) energy. The carrier of male energy (Yang) should take on the greatest manly ascribes. His essence is genuine mindfulness and steadiness. The conveyor of female energy (Yin) should remind female ascribes, like imperativeness, attachment to feelings, and disposition to change. Hence, in Tantra, utilization of sensuality is an instrument to rise above. Ladies are attempting to turn out to be more "ladylike" and men more "manly." In Tantra, the male body is full of Yang energy for the most part, and the female body carries Ying energy. They are opposite energies that attract each other, yet, together, they are balancing the universe. The method of the Tao is consistently a path looking for balance, which is possible to achieve only with the harmonization of the outer Yin and yang (the woman and the man) and the inner Yin and yang (in every lover). The outcome acquired is called "Twofold Elevation."

~ CHAPTER 4 ~
# Tantric Yoga

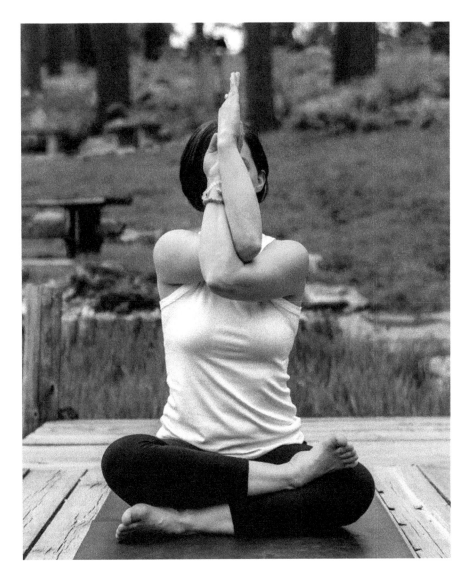

In the past chapters, I introduced the two main branches of tantra: the white tantra and the red tantra (or right and left hand). As already mentioned, the white tantra is a solo path based on yoga and meditation, while the red tantra is based on sexual practices to perform as a couple. They both lead to achieving liberation, but either of them will make you work on different skills and objectives.

The white tantra will help you build more consciousness about yourself and your body, while the red tantra will lead you to create a deeper bond with your partner. While the western neotantra may infer otherwise, the two paths should cooperate to facilitate the final achievement. Chose to walk only one of those paths will make your final goal much more challenging to achieve. Learning Tantric Yoga can make you a better lover, and tantric sex is the opportunity to know more about yourself with the support of your partner.

For this reason, I want to apply in this book some practices for both paths. This chapter will talk about some yoga and breating practices that you exercise in solo, while from the next one, we'll get more in detail about your tantric sexual experience. If you want to get to the hot part sooner, feel free to skip this chapter, but if you are willing to bring your tantric sex to the highest level, you should practice regularly the exercises suggested.

4.1 TANTRIC YOGA POSITIONS

Yoga is an ancient form of exercise based on *asana* (body postures), meditation, and breathing. This kind of workout will help you build flexibility, strength and it's also an efficient technique for relaxation. Tantric yoga is a form of yoga aligned with Tantra. While tantric and classic yoga share most of their meditation techniques and body position, the main difference is the perception of the body. From a classical yoga perspective, the body is inferior because it belongs to the material world. Instead, in tantric perception, material and spiritual are both parts of the creation and treated at the same level. In conclusion, on a practical level, there is no difference between the two; the only difference is purely theoretical. Therefore, as long as you love your body, you perform tantric yoga when doing this kind of exercise.

The reasons why you should perform yoga in Tantra are both physical and spiritual. First, this kind of exercise helps you build stamina and flexibility that you will need for tantric sex. Last but not least, it will help you set up the correct mindset for Tantra, teaching you how to be relaxed and how to manipulate your breathing for the best living. I selected some exercises that, in my experience, are the most helpful for tantric sex. Of course, you can perform them on your own, but if you are a beginner, my suggestion is to follow a class or find someone to show you the correct posture in performing them. Be aware that doing yoga is a healthy practice, but if you have some particular conditions like pregnancy or circular vascular disease is better that you should ask your doctor's opinion before doing yoga.

1. COBRA POSE – BHUJANGASAMA

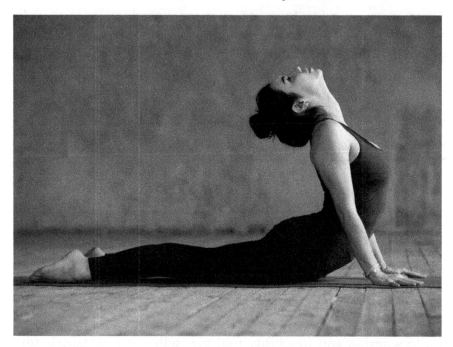

To perform this position, start lying down on your stomach, legs extended, and the toes are pointing straight back and the top of your feet, thighs and pubis firmly into the floor. Spread your hands on the ground under the shoulders and push your torso up. On inhalation, lift your chest off the floor and straighten your arms. Lift the pubis toward the navel and narrow the hips points. When inhaling, your shoulders are moving back, opening your chest. Your shoulders should stay relaxed and the base of your neck soft, while your buttocks are firm but not harden.

Keep this position from 10-30 seconds, breathing easily. After you fully exhale, relaxing your body and going down with your torso. Bend your elbows a little as your chest gets closer to the floor Repeat this sequence from 5 to 10 times. At the end of this practice, you should feel much more light and relaxed!

2. DOWNWARD-FACING DOG – ADHO MUKHA SVANASANA

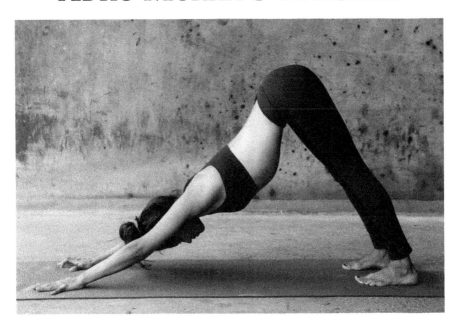

Start this pose in an all-fours position, with the hands slightly forward your shoulders and spread your fingers. Firmly press your hands applying the pressure on the edge of the palms and creating a suction cup in the middle (this status of your hands is called Hasta Bandha). Lift your hips up to bring yourself into an upside-down V pose. In the beginning, keep your knees a bit bent when you adjust your back. Your Shoulders should blade down along the spine, and the base of your neck should stay relaxed. Maintaining your spine stretched, "walk your dog" by alternating bending and straightening your knees.

With each exhalation, root down firmly through your hands; with each subsequent inhalation, send your hips back and up even more. Hold for anywhere from a few breaths to a few minutes, then release. For this position, remember to focus more to keep length in the spine than straight legs, so it's ok to keep your keens a bit bent if you need to feel more comfortable.

3. SUPINE SPINAL TWIST – SUPTA MATSYENDRASAN

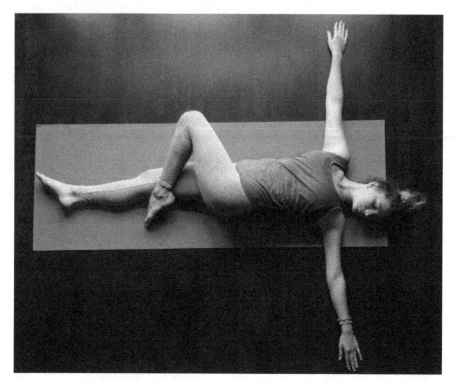

The Supine Spinal Twist stretches the back muscles and realigns and lengthens the spine giving more flexibility and endurance to the subject. Start lying down on your back and bring your arms in a T position, with the palms facing down. Next, bend your right knee over the left side of your body, twisting the spine and low back. Once in this position, use your left hand to push your right knee against the floor; you should feel your thigh and lower back stretching. Your gaze should look in the opposite direction of your knees or toward the ceiling. Keep your shoulders flat to the floor when twisting your body. Keep this position for 6-10 breaths before repeating it with the other side.

4. WARRIOR 1 – VIRABHADRASANA I

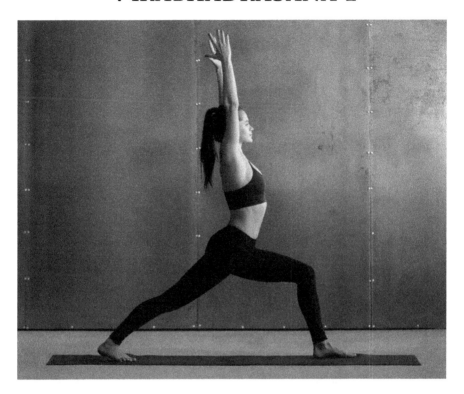

There are three variations for the Warrior Pose, and each of them can be performed to improve your tantric sex. I chose this one because it's ideal for stretching your muscles, and it also helps tone your thighs and butt. It will also improve your stamina and endurance that are always helpful for tantric love.

Start this position standing up straight. Then step your right foot back approximately 45° inward, while your front knee bend at 90° or slightly more. Next, straight your spins and drop your shoulders back while you raise your arms above your head. Your left leg should stay strong as you hold this position for 30 seconds or so. To release, unbend your front knee, centering the torso, and bring your arms down slowly. Repeat the pose bringing back your left leg this time.

5. Plow pose – Halasana

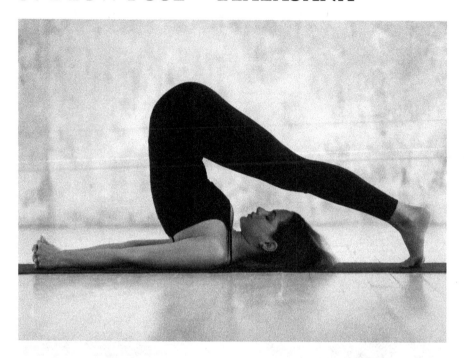

Halasana or Plow (or plough) Pose is an inverted asana that stretches back and shoulders. This pose relaxes the nervous system and relieves stress and fatigue. Consider that this exercise is not a straightforward pose, and you may not get it right at the first attempt. The difficulty level is medium-hight, so it's better if you practice with the previous ones if you are a beginner, and for the first time, it's better if you check with someone that you are in the correct position.

To accomplish this pose, start lying flat on your back with the arms on your sides, hands with palms down, and then extend your legs. When inhaling, use your abdominal muscles to lift your hips and legs. Bring your torso perpendicular to the floor. Keeping your legs extended, slowly lower your toes until touching the floor. If you are struggling to touch the floor, don't worry, you just need some practice; put your toes as lower as you can, keeping the legs extended, and support your back with your hands. If you can reach the floor, then extend your arms and interlace your fingers, pressing your upper arms firmly into the floor. To have this position done correctly:

1. Your Torso is perfectly perpendicular to the floor
2. The legs are extended straight as much as you can
3. There is some space between your chin and the chest and softens your throat. Your eyes should gaze down toward your cheeks.

Once reached the position, hold the pose for up to five minutes. To release, support your backs when returning your legs. Move slowly when rolling down, and if you need, you can bend your knees.

This pose is perfect for letting out your stress, and it's a good exercise for your stamina. It will help you to have better endurance and a relaxed mind.

~ CHAPTER 5 ~
# Breathing

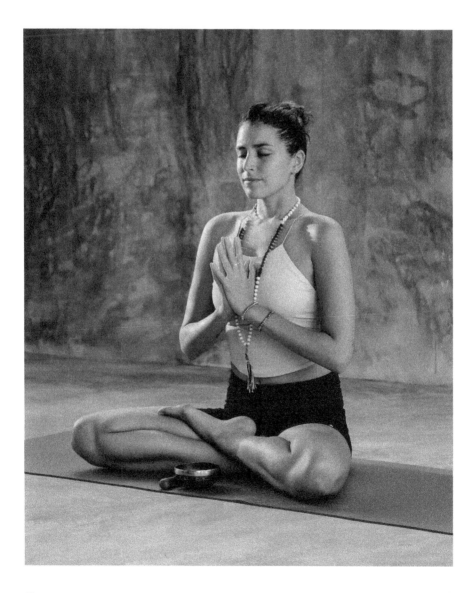

Breathing is an action that comes naturally, and most of the time, people don't even think about it. However, we learn to deal with breath since we get into the world. Without it, we wouldn't be able to stay alive.

Unfortunately, from a very young age, we begin to limit our breath. Remember when your parents screamed at you when you were too loud and too full of energy? We have grown up thinking that being energetic and noisy could cause us trouble, so we soon adjusted our breath to keep it shallow and quiet.

We empower our body with energy through breathing, but this is not necessarily positive; it can also be negative energy. We rarely think about it (or we don't think about it at all), but how we breathe affects our mood and spirit.

You don't have to believe my word; we can do a quick experiment just now. First, try to take a shallow and short breath; don't you feel small and maybe a bit off? Sometimes when I do it, I can perceive a veil of sadness to which I cannot attribute an origin. Now, try again with a deep and long breath. You have to breathe with your chest and not your stomach. Don't you feel much better? More energized and in control?

With breath, we can regulate our mood and recharge our bodies. In Tantra, mastering the breath is the most efficient way to access your chakra and elevate your spirit to illumination.

I suggest using this technique even in everyday life. From now on, try to pay attention to your breathing and if you feel tired and stressed, take a minute to breathe deeply and recharge your body. Your troubles and issues won't change depending on your breathing, but your perspective will.

5.1 Tantra Breathing & Pranayama

Pranayama is the practice adopted in yoga that focuses on controlling the breath. *Prana* is the Sanskrit word meaning "life energy" while *yama* means "control"; so, the whole world pranayama means "control of life energy," and sometimes you can see it also translated as "extension of breath." The ancient yogis recognized how breathing was essential for our body to survive. So, they practiced some techniques to regulate breathing, releasing stress, and increasing physical and mental health.

In tantric sex, breath is essential to connect with another person. If you want to synchronize with your partner (and since you are doing tantric sex, you do want), you must match your breaths. Try to inhale and exhale together; you need to do it intensely and remember to use your chest and not your belly. Breath is like the rhythm of life, and if you are connected with breath, you are dancing together.

Breathing is one of the manners in which Tantra varies from different kinds of sex. With tantric breathing, you center around your accomplice's breathing. Once in a while, it's simply staying there and allowing your bodies to move with each other.

When you practice breathing techniques, stay focused on your respiration. In this status, your mind might move to other matters; it is not simple, but you will be able to master your thoughts after some practice. You have to keep thinking that your current center is breathing with your partner, and nothing else has to interfere.

Keep your thoughts far from the orgasm too. At this point, you don't have to stress yourself about the result. If you relax and stay connected with your partner, the rest will come naturally. Enjoy the moment and work on giving a fun, vivid involvement to the individual you're offering yourself.

Breath is the focal core of all Tantra, and breathing is a way to help free the brain, body, and spirit. At the point when you center around your breathing, you'll feel the sensations significantly more intense, and you'll feel more joyful too.

Achieving the perfect synchronization with your partner through breath may sound easy, but it's more complicated than it seems.

Usually, you're on different frequencies, yet the reflective idea of breathing, performed by you and your partner, considers both of you to remain on a similar frequency and thus, build a more profound connection.

5.2 BREATHING TECHNIQUES

Before introducing some pranayama lessons, I want to provide a few breathing exercises that you can perform to improve the connection with your partner.

Calm Breathing

Calm breathing, sometimes called diaphragmatic breathing, is a technique that helps you slow down your breathing when feeling stressed or anxious. This technique allows you to dominate your feelings and overcome anxiety, but it does require some practice to apply it correctly. All breathing techniques require your body to be straight and sitting upright because this posture increases the capacity of your lungs to fill with air. To perform this technique, sit straight, relax your shoulders and take a slow breath through your nose; you must inhale using your diaphragm or abdomen for about 4 seconds. Next, hold your breath for 1 or 2 seconds, then exhale slowly through the mouth for about 4 seconds. Wait a couple of seconds before repeating. If you want to practice with this technique, do about 6-8 breathing cycles every day. Breathing to your nose is a technique used to awake the Ajna Chakra.

Active Cycle of Breathing Technique (ACBT)

This technique is a 3 phase cycle that helps clear mucus from the lungs.

The first phase is **Breathing control**. Like in the previous exercise, sit straight and relax your shoulders. Next, take a gentle breath inhaling through your nose, and exhale slowly through your mouth using the lower part of your chest. To help yourself to improve the execution, you can put one hand on your stomach as you breathe. If it's difficult for you to exhale with an open mouth, you can purse your lips together to create backpressure in the airways that stents the airway open longer. Repeat breathing control for five breaths before moving forward. This phase helps you to relax your airways.

The second phase is the **Chest expansion exercise**. Place your hands onto your ribs cage, then take a long and deep breath in through the nose. Hold your breath for one-two seconds before releasing it with a long gentle breath out through the mouth. During this phase, you should focus on the movements of your ribs that are contracting and expanding during the exercise. Again, you can exhale with an open mount or pursing your lips together to make it easier. Repeat this phase for five breaths.

The last phase is called the **Forced expiration technique**. This phase forces the mucus out of your lungs, so you don't need this phase for relaxation, but you can use it to clear your airways. For this last part, you can mimic steaming a window or a mirror; if you want, you can use your hand in front of you to visualize one of the two. First, take a breath in through the nose, and then open your mouth and huff the air out. You can perform this one in two ways: take a long breath in and a short and quick exhalation, or inhale quickly and breath out slowly. Repeat five times, then complete the cycle with a cough to clear your lungs.

4-7-8 breath

This technique works amazingly to relieve physical and mental pressure. It is suggested to execute this breathing exercise while facing your partner; this will help to synchronize your breaths. Before starting the breathing pattern, adopt a comfortable sitting position and place the tip of the tongue on the tissue right behind the top front teeth. You can do this with your accomplice while holding each other's hand, focusing only on your breathing.

Breathing cycle:
- Breath in for 4 seconds
- Hold your breath for 7 seconds
- Exhale for 8 seconds
- Repeat the cycle four times

5.3 Pranayamas – some effective breathing exercises

Pranayama is a way of reaching higher states of consciousness and is an excellent practice to keep the body and mind healthy. In this section, I selected three of the most effective pranayama techniques. They will help you to calm your mind and to find focus while you are breathing.

When you practice yoga and breathing techniques for the first time, you should do it with the guidance of a knowledgeable teacher. Do not attempt any breathing and yoga exercise if you have a respiratory condition or pregnant without consulting your doctor first. Stop the exercise if you become faint or dizzy. If you have any medical concerns, talk with your doctor before practicing yoga and breathing techniques.

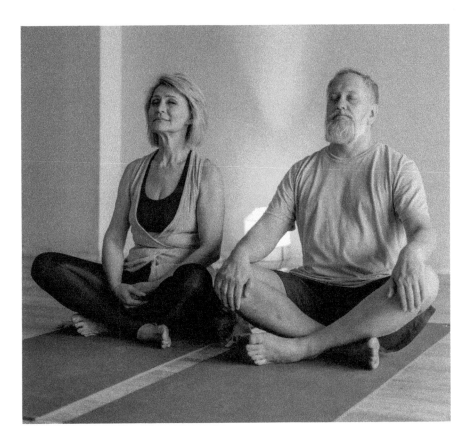

Bhastrika Pranayama – Bellows Breath

Bhastrika, or "bellows breath," is a traditional breathing exercise in yoga that helps to increase *prana* (energy) in your body. This technique helps to remove excess congestion in the lungs and brighten the mind. If you haven't tried this method before, you can stop in the middle and pause from 15 up to 30 seconds. Make sure to listen to your body during the practice. Bellows breathing is a safe practice, but if you feel light-headed in any way, take a pause for a few minutes while breathing naturally. Then, when the discomfort passes, try another round of bellows breathing, slower and less intense.

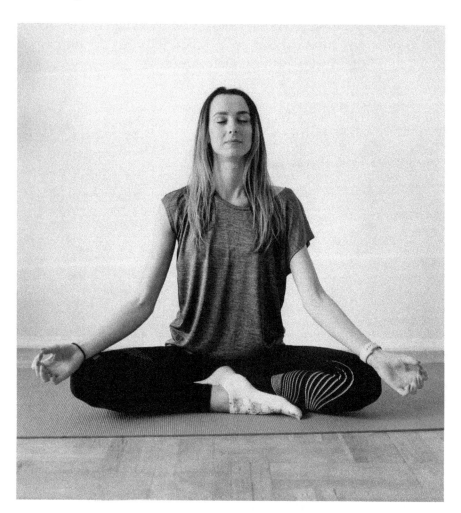

To perform Bhastrika:

- Sit up tall, relax your shoulders.
- Take a few deep breaths in and out from your nose.
- With each inhale, expand your belly fully as you breathe.
- As you breathe out, feel the pelvic floor lifting, which helps bring blood flow to that region.
- Keep your head, neck, shoulders, and chest still while your belly moves in and out.
- After 27 rounds of Bhastrika, take a full breath in and hold, retaining the breath.
- With your hands, clamp the abdominal muscles at the lower abdomen and, as you keep the breath, lift and lower the head gently 3-5 times.
- Release the clamp and breath normally.

You can attempt this technique with your partner facing each other and try to copy each other's moves, but if one of you is in discomfort, try to slow it down.

Nadi Shodhana and Anulom Vilom Pranayama

Known as *Alternate nostril breathing*, it's a technique used for relaxation. This technique involves holding one nostril closed with your thumbs while inhaling. Then, keeping the other nostril closed while exhaling. This practice is ideal for balancing the breath, and if done regularly, it can improve circulation and calm the nervous system.

To perform *Anulom Vilom*:

- Sit in Padmasan (sitting with your legs crossed but both your feet are on your thighs) or if you feel more comfortable, sit with your legs crossed. Rest your hands and your knees and relax your shoulders.
- Close the right nostril with the right thumb while inhaling from the left one.
- Breath in expanding your lungs as much as possible.
- When switching from inhalation to exhalation, remove

the thumb from your right nostril and use your middle finger to close your left nostril. Then exhale, releasing all the air in your lungs.
- Repeat this process for five minutes keeping your focus on your breath.

Once you get used to the *Anulom Vilom*, you can proceed with the next level, which is called *Nadhi Sodhana*. This technique is very similar to the previous one but with two differences. This time, you inhale through the left nostril and breath out through the right. Additionally (and most important), you need to hold your breath for a minute or so between your inhalation and exhalation. Repeat this cycle for 3 or 5 minutes.

As the Anulom Vilom, the Nadhi Sodhana helps relax your mind and body, and it's an ideal exercise for a healthy heart.

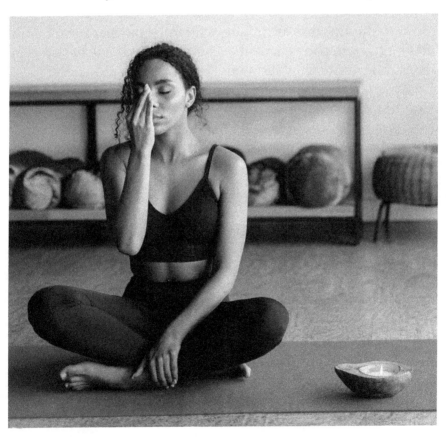

Ujjayi Pranayama

Ujjayi Pranayama is one technique that helps to relax your brain and warm the body. The Sanskrit word ujjayi means "conquer," "being victorious," but because of the sound created when performed correctly, it is also referred to as "ocean breath." Ujjayi encourages the full expansion of the lungs while slightly contracting your throat and breathe through your nose. When practicing Ujjayi Pranayama, be careful not to tighten your throat.

To perform Ujjayi Pranayama:
- Sit in the Easy Pose (or Sukhasana pose - sitting on the floor crossing your legs and having your back straight). Relax your shoulders and close your eyes.
- Let your mouth drop open slightly. Inhale and exhale deeply through your mouth. When exhaling, softly whisper the sound "ahhh" while slightly contracting the back of your throat.
- When you got comfortable with your exhalation, try to maintain the constriction of the throat even when you breathe in. You should notice an "ocean waves" sound coming from your breath if you do this properly.
- When you get comfortable with this breathing and position, you can try to close your mouth and breathe only through your nose. Keep the constriction in your throat like you were doing when the mouth was open. The "ocean sound" should keep coming from your breath. When you get comfortable breathing through your nose, direct the air over your vocal cords, across the back of your throat.
- Concentrate on the sound of your breath; it should be soft and gentle. When breathing in, fill your lungs to their fullest expansion and empty them when you exhale.

Start practicing Ujjayi for five minutes per day; for more profound meditation, increase your time to 15 minutes. Once you get familiar with this breathing technique; also, you can apply Ujjayi while doing yoga.

~ CHAPTER 6 ~
Preparation

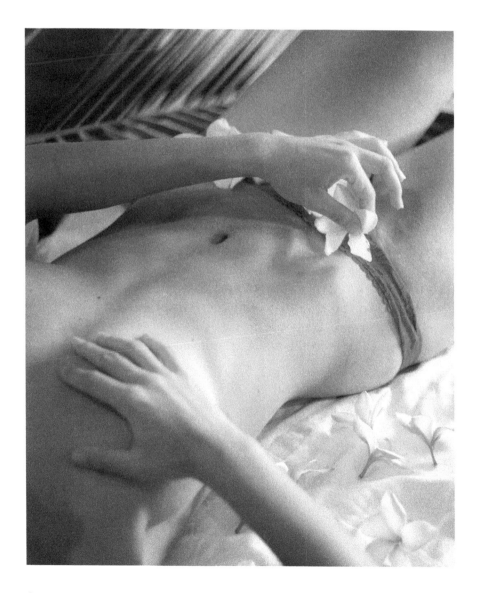

So far, we came across the theoretical part of Tantra, exploring its meaning and its history. But the best part has yet to come because, finally, we are going to learn some practical techniques. It should be clear until now how important is sex in Tantra, but before mastering the "act of love," you need to learn some tactics that will help you and your partner get the most delightful experience.

First, it is essential to focus on your body and the development of sexual activity to advance energy flow.
Secondly, communication during love can't be denied or interrupted. In tantric sex, one shouldn't hesitate to communicate their pleasure at 100%.

At long last, breath is also an excellent alliance to accomplishing satisfaction. You can use some breathing exercises to perform along the whole circle of sexual affectivity for better outcomes.

Talk with your partner

Before starting, ensure that you and your accomplice both want to attempt this. Tantric sex can be a great experience, but it won't work if one or both of you have some hesitation. Keep in mind, it takes two to tango, and that goes for tantric sex as well. Going for tantric sex is an experience that you have to do together. If you're keen on doing it, you need to ensure that your accomplice is in the same spot as you are.

The vast majority don't understand that this is something that the partner may not be ready for yet. You may think beginning immediately is a good thought but forcing your partner will only add pressure on your relationship. Tantra is a process that takes time and preparation, so don't rush it. You need cooperation and synchronization for doing it, and starting with the wrong foot won't be beneficial.

If you're rehearsing tantric sex, yet your partner is not, you won't be able to coordinate because the two of you would move to a different rhythm. If you don't synchronize, one will encounter orgasm early and try to slow down, while the other will rush to catch up. With this dysfunctionality, you won't be able to be one and the other, like Shiva and Shakti, so you'll never reach the greatest pleasure.

Anyway, it shouldn't be challenging to convince your partner. Tantra is an experience that brings to the couple more intimacy and energy. Whatever is the status of your relationship, Tantra is the better way to spice it up. So, all considered, if you open your mind to this path, it will take you to places where you have never been before.

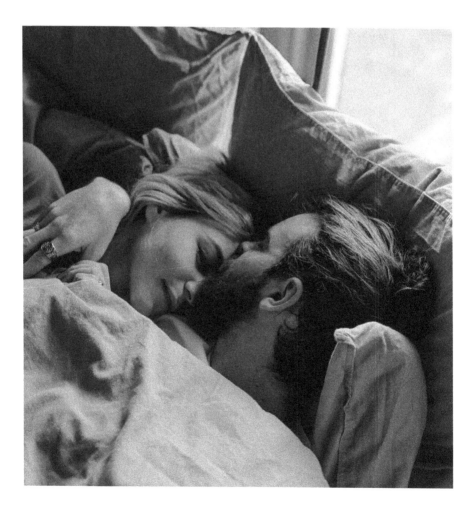

Prepare your body

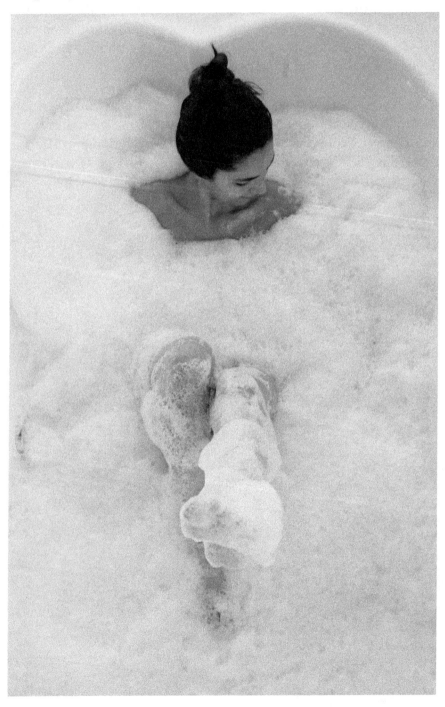

Preparing your body for the Tantra experience is an excellent practice because it will help you relax and recharge your energy. It can also be a grand affair if you and your partner decide to do it together.

There are several options to prepare your body: doing yoga or meditation, practice your breath, showering, and massaging your body. These alternatives have the purpose of taking you to relaxation and losing the tension accumulated during the day. You don't have to do them all; pick up what fits you most.

Although yoga, meditation, and breathing exercise should be considered hobbies rather than actions to apply just before lovemaking. You can use them before sex if they make you feel regenerated, but I recommend doing something that can make you feel good and recharged.

What I like to do most for my preparation is having a long bath. The warm water and the scents help me recharge my spirit, and when I do it with my partner, I feel more connected with him because I am sharing one of the experiences that I like most.

Preparing the body with your partner is not only a great way to build more intimacy, but you can use this situation to do things that would be difficult to do alone. For instance, you can ask your partner to make you a massage, so you don't have to stress out for doing this yourself, and you can fully enjoy the relaxation.

When you get ready together, I suggest taking turns. Allow your partner to help you to relax, let them do a massage, or ask them to refresh your back, and when they have fished, it's your turn to return the favor. During each turn, don't be afraid to give the feedback that you need to. It's ok to tell your partner what they should do better, which will help them give you what you want.

Communication

Agreeing to initiate the tantra path together is not the only step in communication. It may sound redundant in the relationship, but this aspect is a valuable key for tantric sex.

If you want to achieve the highest orgasm, you need to let your partner know what you like so that they can give you the best pleasure. In the same way, you need to listen to the other attendant's lead to provide them the highest gratification.

Don't wait until the end of the session to explain your needs. You have to keep the communication going at every stage of the sexual encounter.

Prepare the atmosphere

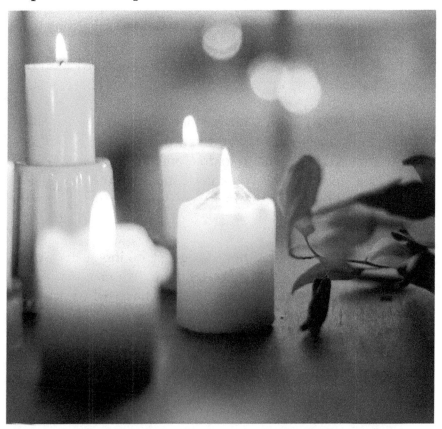

Even if this may sound secondarily important, setting the room where you will share the act of love is a great tip to make you feel more confident and get in the right mood.

Make sure that the room has everything you need to make yourself and your partner comfortable. Prepare the bed, or use a soft carpet if you prefer. Check that you have enough pillows, you don't necessarily have to use them, but it's good to have them around if you feel you need them. They are also helpful allies in case you want to adjust your position if you feel uncomfortable.

Feel free to add candles, flowers, and petals if you think they will help to set the atmosphere, but make sure that they won't be in the way during the performance. Another essential element is light. I don't recommend having tantric sex in the darkness because it will negatively affect your senses and impact your ability to synchronize with your partner.

For tantric sex, the best illumination is a soft light. You can use the lamps for the bedsides or, even better, turning some candles on. If you decide to use the candles, don't use too many of them, a couple would be enough, and please, be careful to put them in a safe place.

Possibly, avoid the colored light, especially the red one. It may look sensual, but red is the most inadequate color for relaxation. This suggested type of illumination, aside from being more romantic, helps concentrate on what is in front of us without disrupting the flow of energies.

The scent is also a valuable component in your room. Most people usually underestimate the power of smell, but it's a valid stimulator for love and relaxation. Scented candles may help to cover this point too, or you can make use of incense. If you are missing both, using some perfume to lightly scent the linens will do just fine.

Diet

In general, a healthy diet is suitable for longer life. This component is also suggested for Tantra because it will help you stay in the right shape to achieve advanced sexual positions. Sure, you don't have to follow a specific diet if you don't want to. And I also don't recommend trying any advanced position before you and your partner have built enough experience to move to a higher step. Anyway, my suggestion is to have a light meal when you are approaching the tantra event. Also, make sure to give your body enough time to digest and enough calories to support the performance. In some ways, it is good to approach the tantric relationship as a sport and provide our bodies with the most suitable nutrients.

Personally, I prefer to have a light meal made of white meats and vegetables and bring some peeled fruit to the room in the case of a long and tiring session.

~ CHAPTER 7 ~
The sensual touch

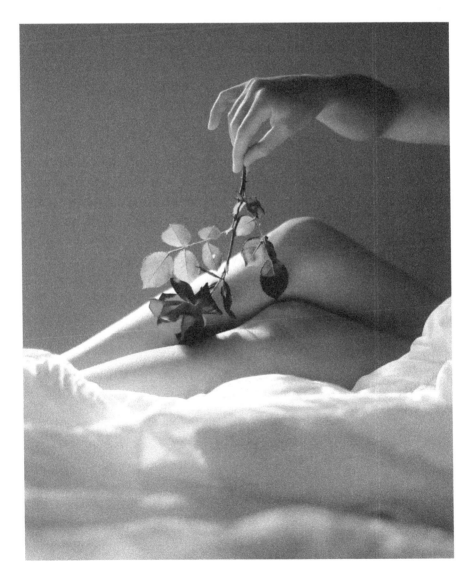

With ordinary sex, tactile sensations are predominant, and the other four senses tend to take second place. It may sound odd, but most practices of tantric sex don't even require the subjects to use their hands to touch each other, but that won't obstacle in achieving great pleasure; instead, it exalts the fusion of the spirits.

Tantric sex isn't only a little influx of enjoyment but a profound and hypnotizing wave of pleasure brought by the orgasm. It's astounding how few changes applied in sex may take to different outcomes. Tantric sex doesn't generally involve much contact, nor does it need to consider making loud noises. Tantric sex is mainly based on using the balancing and expansion of internal energies to achieve absolute pleasure.

IMPORTANT: The massage techniques that I will explain to you next shouldn't be applied before the tantric sex. If you do so, you may get excited too soon, and you and your partner may get to an orgasm even before the actual sexual activity has started. The tantric massages that I am sharing with you are not a companion of the actual fusion but are techniques that you can use to build intimacy with your partner. These can be valid alternatives for a romantic evening to spend together, and they can give a sip of the benefits that Tantra can bring in your life and relationship.

7.1 How to Touch Your Shiva

In contrast to an ordinary sensual massage, the tantric massage of the penis and lingam it's not just meant to provoke your partner's physical orgasm. Instead, with this massage technique, you want to slowly awaken this critical erogenous zone and the powerful sexual energy hidden in it. Here's how to perform a tantric massage on your man.

First, it is essential to create a distraction-free environment where you can let yourself be absorbed entirely in the moment. For this reason, remove any irritating and disturbing element, i.e., clocks or any font of noise or undesired light. Another reason for eliminating clocks from the room is that this massage can take a long time. We are not interested in keeping track of time but only in the sensations we are experiencing at that moment. As suggested before, you can light up the room with scented candles and incense to make the atmosphere even more engaging.

Start the foreplay as you usually would, touch your partner until sexual arousal. Try to involve all the senses. Strip slowly to engage his sense of sight. Caress his body to engage the sense of touch. Let him feel the scent of your skin and the taste of your kisses. Bring him to arousal with words or moans of pleasure Before starting the authentic tantric massage, it is essential to know how your partner reacts to the stimulation of his different erogenous zones. Try to understand which are more sensitive and which are less, exploring not only the penis but also the perineum, the scrotum, and the inner thigh.

Oil is a fundamental element in Tantric massage. I recommend that you use sweet almond, coconut, or jojoba oil to enhance your sexual experience. Another essential element while performing the lingam (penis) massage is breathing. Both partners should use the *Bliss Breath* technique that consists of a series of deep breaths. First, inhale and focus on receiving the energy of arousal and pleasure from your partner. Then, exhale and focus on sending them loving energy. Continue to use this breathing technique during the massage.

Oil the shaft of the penis and the testicles. Start by slowly sliding your hands up and down the thighs. Wait until your partner feels relaxed and his body got used to your touch.

Move on the testicles. Gently, slowly massage them. Remember to keep using the Bliss Breath. Feel free to softly use your fingernails or slightly pull the testicles to provide some extra stimulation. During this massage, do not neglect the pubic bone in the front, the inner part of the thighs, and the perineum (the area between the testicles and the anus).

When you feel your partner aroused enough, start working on the shaft of the penis. During this process, it is essential to experiment with different approaches. Variety is the key to achieving the perfect orgasm. Here some ideas:

- Vary your grip from harder to lighter.
- Vary the speed from slow to fast. Then, you can tease your lover, building up from slow to fast and going back to slow again.
- Alternate strokes with one and two hands. Also, when you work with one hand, you can alternate left and right.
- Add some twisting in your strokes from time to time.
- Alternate deep strokes, that start from the base of the penis until the head, and short and rapid strokes.
- When playing with two hands, the bottom hand can move up and down while the top hand can add a twisting motion on the tip of the penis.

It is important not to let your partners come too quickly. Instead, try to keep him on the verge of orgasm. This is not an easy task; it requires some practice in reading his body language. Some indicators that an orgasm is imminent are changes in their breathing and involuntary micro muscle contractions. When you see them at the edge, pull back on what you are doing, or just slow it down and remind them to breathe and ride the wave of orgasmic feelings they are experiencing.

Start to stimulate the prostate (externally). To find the prostate (also called sacred spot), look for an indentation between the testicles and the anus. This spot has typically the size of a pea. Lightly press the area with your fingers or knuckles or use a circular massage motion. Let your partner guide you in order to apply the correct pressure. This spot is very sensitive. Try not to press too hard. Especially in the beginning, it is a good idea to ask your partner how they feel.

If your partner wants to try some anal play, you can stimulate the sacred spot internally. But, first, ensure that both your fingers and the area are well lubricated. Then, start massaging the outside of the anus in a slow circular motion. This will help loosen up the anal muscles making easy the penetration. Next, slowly insert the tip of your finger and move it until you feel minimal resistance. Remember to keep adding oil since the anus, unlike the vagina, is unable to lubricate itself. Once your partner feels comfortable, start to search for the prostate, usually situated 2 to 3 inches inside the anus, closer to the anterior wall of the rectum.

Once you reach the prostate, you can massage it moving your finger side to side or apply gentle pressure. Ask your partner how he feels so that you can adjust the movement based on how he feels.

To end the massage, you can allow your partner to climax or move on to sex.

7.2 How to Touch Your Shakti

One of the most famous tantric massages for ladies is the Yoni massage. If you have forgotten, the word *yoni* is the Sanskrit word used for the female genital organ.

Some allude to the vagina as a "consecrated sanctuary." This is because the vagina is an erogenous zone with the right to be investigated in an unexpected way, symbolizing the entrance to paradise.

Yoni has a primary role in Tantra. If you remember from the chapter describing the story of this sacred path, Tantra was born with the image of the female figure as its focus, and, of course, the vagina has the most crucial role in this part.

The fundamental objective of the Yoni massage is to make the lady profoundly excited and experience sensations that she has never experienced before. Also, the massage performed by men's fingers further expands the level of intimacy between the couple. The accomplice of the massage is classified "giver," to give the lady all the pleasure she merits and ought to anticipate nothing consequently.

Remember that I don't recommend using any of these massages before making love since these techniques accelerate the coming of the orgasm. If you decide to use this massage, you must consider that, if you do it properly, your female partner should reach the orgasm (and even having more than one), and you'll probably end without sex.

But, if you decide to try this massage, I am sure your lady will be very grateful. So, get ready to learn the Yoni massage procedure!

Set up the room. As mentioned in the previous chapters, be sure the light is right, and there are no distractions in the room.

The lady should lie on her back in a comfortable position with a pillow under her hips, the knees up, and the feet on the ground.

Synchronize your breathing. For the Yoni massage to work, it is significant that your breathing is synchronized. Try to inhale and exhale out together, keeping your breathing regular and slow. It is advisable to use the Bliss Breath; this technique consists of a series of deep breaths. First, inhale and focus on receiving the energy of arousal and pleasure from your partner. Then, exhale and focus on sending them loving energy. Continue to use this breathing technique during the massage.

Before starting with the real massage we want to do a short warm-up. Oil is a fundamental element; I recommend using sweet almond, coconut, or jojoba oil to enhance your sexual experience. Start to apply some oil on the belly and gently massage the area. Don't neglect the rib cage between the breasts and the lower abdomen. Use slow and delicate movements until you reach the breasts and the areolae. Don't touch the nipples yet until it is not clear that your lady is ready for it!

When you both think it is the right moment, start to tease the nipples alternating between circle movements and light pinching. Then, when you feel that your partner is aroused enough, it's time to perform the real yoni massage. You can apply various techniques to stimulate your partner; feel free to mix them based on your partner's feelings.

1. **Circles:** With this technique, we want to stimulate the external tip of the clitoris with a circular motion of the fingers. You can vary the pressure and the size of the circles based on your partner's reactions.
2. **Push & Pull:** Slide your finger down both sides of the shaft of the clitoris. Most people are more sensitive on one part of the clitoris than another; check your partner's reaction to understand where you should stimulate more.

3. **Tug & Roll:** You grasp the clitoris from the sides and gently pull back and forth with this technique. You can also gently roll the clitoris between your fingers.
4. **Tapping:** You can use one or more fingers to tap the clitoris gently.
5. **G-Spot Massage:** To find the G-Spot, curve your first two fingers like the letter "C" and slowly insert them in the vagina. About an inch or two in, you should feel a slightly ridged area at the top of the vaginal canal, just behind the external clitoris. Slowly stimulate that spot, first with gentle pressure or circle movements and later with a mix of fast and slow strokes.

Remember that the primary goal of Yoni massage is not having an orgasm; it is about feeling waves of pleasure ed eventually have multiple orgasms.

~ CHAPTER 8 ~
Tantric Positions

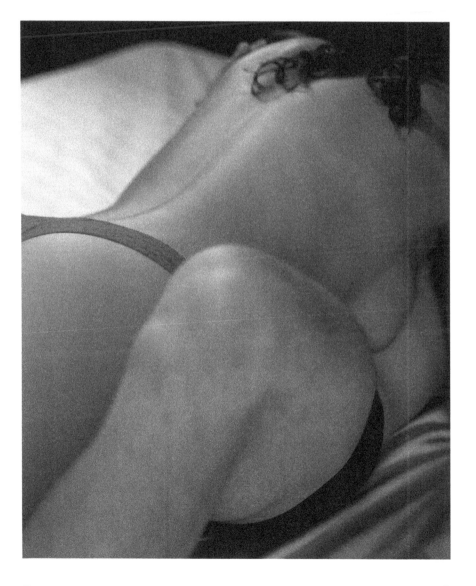

This chapter is probably the one you were waiting for and the reason you bought this book. Now that you have prepared your body and the environment to accomplish the tantric sex, it's time to know some positions that you can try with your partner.

For each technique, I added an indication of its difficulty in performing it. Still, you should consider that the complexity of one position depends on the strength and flexibility of the two subjects. So, finding a tantric position easy or complex is subjective to the couple.

Anyway, when I judged these techniques, I considered that some movements might make you feel more natural and comfortable, while others are more elaborated. So, my suggestion is to start with the easiest ones and escalate to higher levels little by little.

1. YAB YUN

The Yab Yum, even known as the *lotus sex position,* is one of the most common practices in Tantra. The world is the translation of "Father-Mother." The man sits with his legs crossed (called "Easy Pose"), and the lady sits on the gentleman's knees facing him, wrapping her legs around his torso. The hands can go around each other's back, or waist, or shoulders, or you can even move your hand on your partner's chest, feeling their beating.

You can reach this final position slowly, starting both from the "easy pose" (sitting with your legs crossed) facing each other and spending some time watching into each other's eyes and synchronizing your breaths. When you are ready, the lady slowly changes position sitting on his legs and wrapping her legs around his lower back.

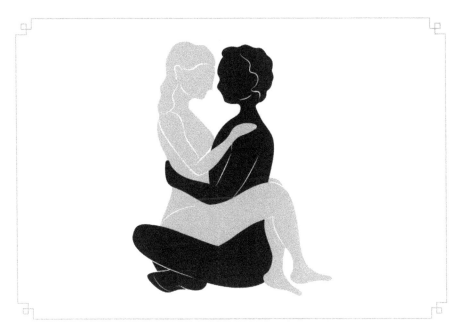

Complexity

While executing the Yab Yum position, you can close your eyes since you are supposed to keep the connection with your partner through the touch and synchronization of your breaths.

In this position, you should feel your bodies exchanging energy. The female power (and the creative life force) rises while the man sits under the woman giving his support as a solid container. Two opposite forces united into one shape.

Hint: Usually, the men don't resist staying in the easy pose for long. You can use some pillows to make him feel more comfortable. He can sit on them or use them under his knees.

2. Sidewinder (Side wind-her)

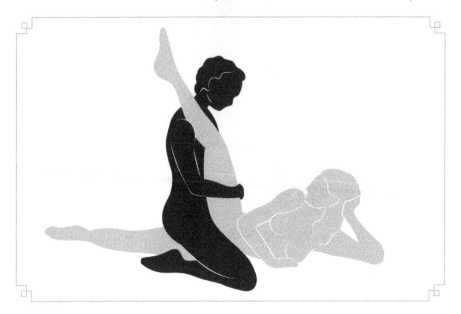

Complexity

The girl should lie on one side and raise the top leg, keeping the bottom one straight on the floor. The gentleman should sit on the bottom lady's thigh, hugging the extended leg on the top; the lady's caff resting on his shoulder.

Hint: Once he is inside her, the man should whirl his hips as he thrusts. With these movements, he'll be able to touch different zones inside the woman's vagina, raising the pleasure to a higher level.

3. PADLOCK

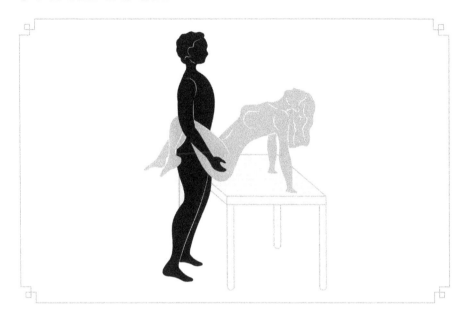

Complexity 🔥 🔥 💧 💧 💧

In this position, the girl sits at the edge of a waist-high piece of furniture, opening her legs and using her arms to support her upper body. Then, the man comes in between the lady's legs, penetrating her, and she wraps her legs around him. For this final shape, this position is also known as *Leg Lock*. Tables and washing machines suit perfectly for this performance. If the man needs added height, he can use some support to stand on it. This position makes it easy for the penetrating partner to stimulate the woman's clitoris.

Hint: With this technique, it's easy for you to keep eye contact. Start this by looking into each other's eyes to increase your affinity, but when it comes, feel free to close your eyes and get lost in the pleasure.

4. Amazing Butterfly

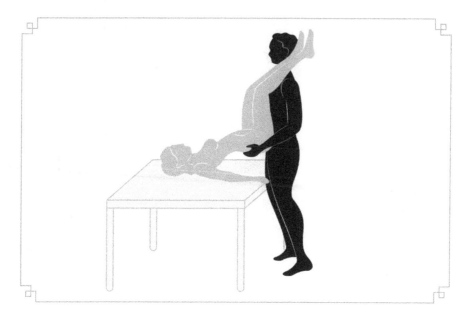

Complexity 🔥🔥🔥🔥🔥

Starting from the padlock position, you can make things a little more challenging. First, the girl should lie on the table and raising her legs, resting her calves on the partner's shoulders. Next, the man should support the lady's back, placing his hands under her hips. With this position, the booty is at the perfect angle while he thrusts.

Hint: In this position, the pelvic tilt gives his penis full access to the vagina exposing female zones that are very sensitive to pleasure. The man should make slow movements and try different pressures to explore what his lady likes most.

5. MERMAID

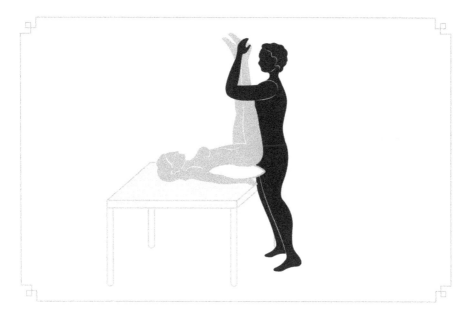

Complexity 🔥🔥🔥 💧 💧

The Mermaid position is another technique that requires medium-high. Very similar to the previous two, the lady lies on her back and raises her legs. But, in the earlier positions, the legs were widely spread apart. For this technique, they need to stay together, like having a long fishtail instead of two legs (which explains the name of this pose).

Hint: To make the Mermaid position more comfortable, make sure that you and your partner's genital are almost at the same level to facilitate the penetration. Also, to avoid reducing his mobility and comfort, the man should avoid bending his knees; instead, he should stand straight. Finally, remember that he can acquire some extra-high using some support if needed.

6. DOUBLE DECKER

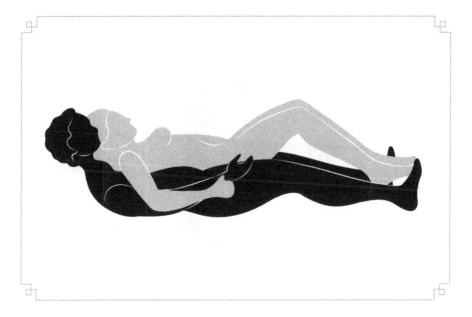

Complexity 🔥 🔥 🔥 🔥 🔥

This position's name comes probably from the popular double-decker buses that became an icon for London, England. During the Double Decker, the two partners lie on their backs, having the lady on top of him. The receiving partner's back on the giver's chest while he penetrates her from behind. Tantric sex rarely allows the men to lie on their back, but this position is an exception since the G-Spot is easy to reach because perfectly aligned with the angle of penetration.

Hint: You can decide to use this technique to penetrate the anus instead of the vagina. In this way, you can try this position with two different variations. For this reason, the Double Decker is recommended for gay or lesbian couples too.

7. Lap Dance

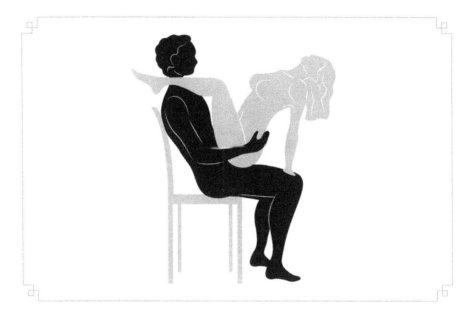

Complexity

The Lap Dance position is a technique where the woman mainly controls the sexual activity while the man can choose to relax and 'enjoy the show' or be a bit more proactive. To perform it, the man must sit on a chair or sofa with the legs wide open. Next, the girl sits on him, guiding his member into the vagina. Then, she should lean backward slightly, placing her hands on his knees. Finally, the lady's legs should extend, resting the ankles on his shoulders.

Hint: To improve the thrusting power, the lady can adjust the weight between the ankles and the hands. The man should tilt his back a little for a better connection, using an angle between 100° and 120° instead of straight at 90°. Also, he can use a pillow to feel more comfortable.

8. G-Force

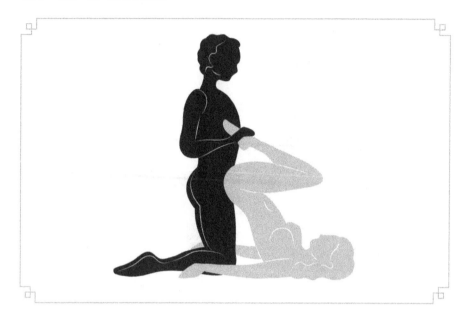

Complexity 🔥🔥🔥🔥🔥

The girl lies down on her back and pulls the knees close to her chest to start this position. Next, the man kneels, pulling her from her hips when penetrating her. Once the partners are connected, the man can move his hands to grab her feet and penetrate. This position is perfect to stimulate her G-Spot and allows the man to be in control. G-Force also allows a reasonable degree of eye contact, and the mane can enjoy the lady's expressions while giving her pleasure.

Hint: For a variation of this position, the lady can place her calves on his shoulders. This new angle of penetration will change the zones stimulated inside her vagina, giving her a new gamma of sensations.

9. WATERFALL

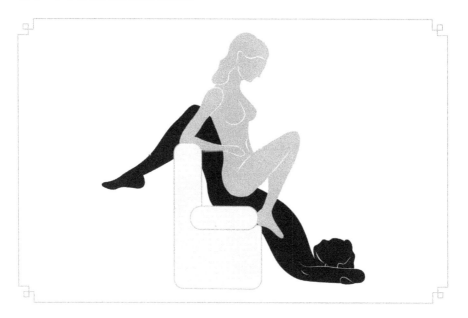

Complexity 🔥 🔥 🔥 🔥 🔥

In the Waterfall is a position the woman is on top. The man lies face up with the head and torso off the edge of the bed and the shoulders resting on the ground. The lady sits then on top of, him leading the penetration. With this technique, the receiving partner is in control, and from her point of view, she can see the companion's reaction. In addition, the blood floating to the head of the gentleman will amplify his sensations.

Hint: You can try this position on the sofa or the armchair, with the giver's legs resting on the backrest.

10. Passion Pretzell

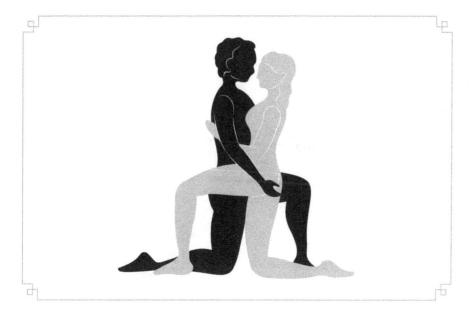

Complexity 🔥 🔥 🔥 🔥 🔥

In this position, you are both kneeling, facing each other. Both of you should place the opposite foot flat on the ground and get closer until penetrating. Then, you and your partner should alternate in leaning forward and backward for thrusting, keeping your lower parts planted to the floor. With this position, male and female roles are equal, two opposite parts completing each other. Use your free arms and hands to build up more intimacy, and remember to keep eye contact.

Hint: It's challenging to maintain this position for a long time; remember to stay as comfortable as possible performing it on a carpet and using pillows. If you start to struggle, consider transitioning into the Yab Yum position to release the tension in your muscles.

11. TUB TANGLE

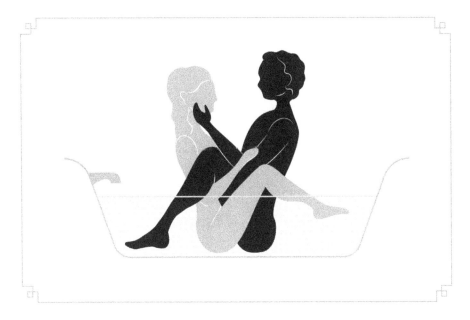

Complexity

What I love about tantric sex is how your surroundings can help to experiment with some techniques, so most of the rooms in the house can be inspiring for trying different experiences. This position is the one to try in the bathtub, facing each other and both of you with the knees bent, keeping the feet planted on the bottom of the bathtub. Once you get into contact, feel free to wrap the legs around your partner's back and link the elbows under each other's knees.

Hint: Since your lips are very close to each other, take this opportunity to exchange passionate kisses and play with your mouths.

12. TORRID TIDAL WAVE

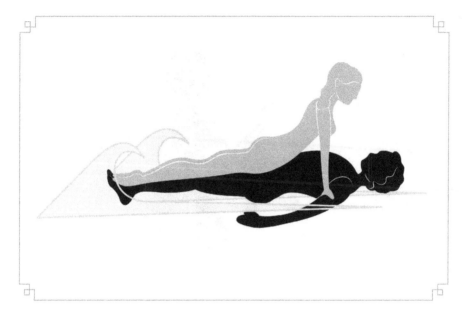

Complexity

The Torrid Tidal Wave is the perfect position to try during a vacation and make you feel like two teenagers. The man lies on his back at the water's edge on a beach, keeping the legs extended and together. The woman lays face-down on him, having the pelvises aligned. Then the lady expands her arms to lift her torso, putting her weight on the hands. In this position, enjoy the waves on your skin; they will amplify your sensations.

Hint: With this technique, the clitoris rubs against the man's pelvic bone. The lady should sporadically clench her butt cheeks tight to increase the feeling of the penis inside her body.

13. GREAT BEE

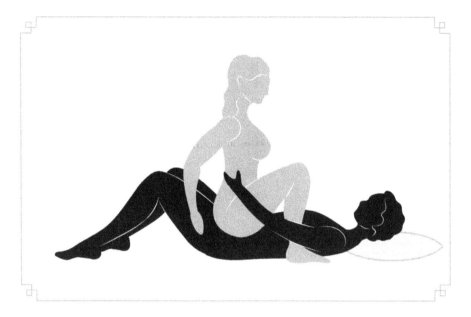

Complexity

For the Great Bee, the man lies down on his back while the lady sits on him in a squat position, having her knees blended to her chest. In this situation, she has absolute control of the tantric sex. Supporting herself with her hands against the lover's thighs, she can perform every movement that she wants, controlling the speed, the penetration, and the frequency.

Hint: When thrusting, I suggest the lady rotate her hips in wide circles. Try also with different pressures on his body to make him feel different intensities.

14. TIME BOMB

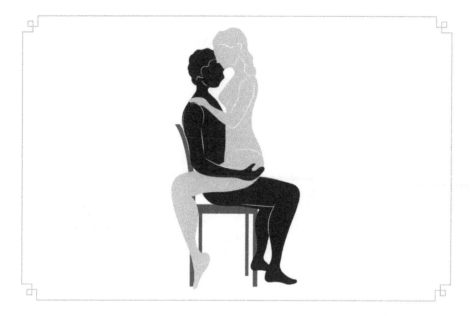

Complexity

In the Time Bomb, the man is sitting on a chair, having his legs relaxed. The woman approaches, facing him and sitting on his erected member; her legs loosened too, having the feet reaching the floor. The arms of both are free, so you can use them to increase your intimacy, like having your hands on each other's chests to adjust your breaths.

Hint: In this position, the woman is in control. When penetrating, do it slowly, inch by inch, to the very end. Then increase the speed gradually to make him feel the different sensations.

15. LOVE TRIANGLE

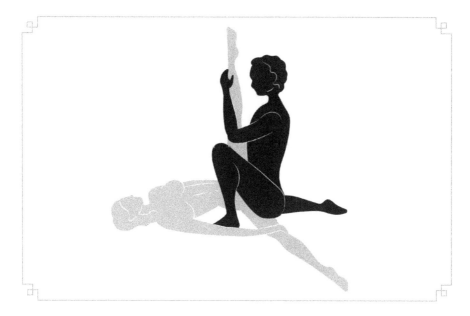

Complexity 🔥 🔥 🔥 🔥 🔥

In the Love Triangle position, the woman lies on her back with the left leg sticking on the floor while the right one is straight up in the air. Having her helping herself with the right hand under the knee, she should stretch her right leg on the side, having it at 90° to her body. If you are akin to geometry, this shape reminds the z-axis in a 3D cartesian coordinate system. Once she is in position, the male partner should crouch at the bottom of her body and start penetrating.

Hint: From this position, the man has free access to the whole vagina. When penetrating, he can rotate his body slightly to try different angulations.

16. ONE PINCER

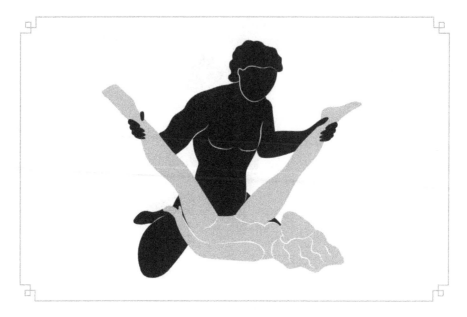

Complexity

The lady lies down on her back with the legs spread wide open in the One Pincer position. The partner kneels in front of her, grabbing her feet and supporting her legs. In this sex experience, the man is in control, but the lady can have some authority too from her bottom position. She can use her free arms to pull the partner's tights to her body, suggesting the speed of the penetration.

Hint: With this position, the man not only can access the vagina freely, but he has free access to the anus as well, in case you want to try this experience too.

17. TILTED MISSIONARY

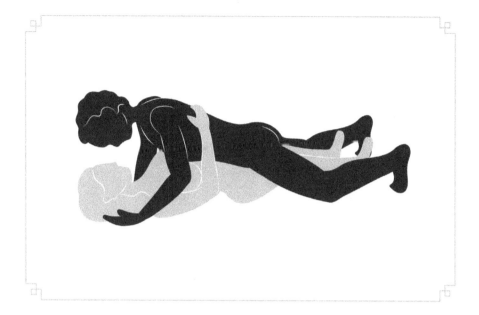

Complexity

There is a reason why some positions are more famous than others. The different techniques that you can apply with the missionary pose allow a better connection between the couple and keep the upper body free enough to build synchronization and look into each other eyes. The lady lies on her back while the man lies on top of her facing each other. For a more comfortable position, the woman can add a pillow under her butt; this will also help to have the vagina more exposed.

Hint: After some time in this position, I suggest the lady moving her legs over the man's shoulders. With this variation, the penetrating part can reach the G-Spot easily and experience some jolts of great pleasure.

18. Snake Trap

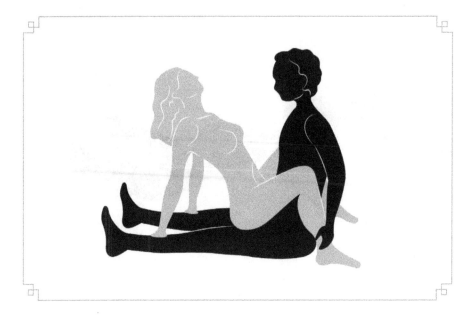

Complexity

The Snake Trap position should be performed in bed or on the floor. The man sits down with his torso straight, and the legs open in a V shape. The lady approaches facing him and sits on him, having the legs in the same shape as the male partner's. The couple is now sitting across from one another, facing each other. The torso should lean backward slightly for both the accomplices, supporting the weight on their hands.

Hint: This position is for shallow penetrations. For better stabilization, grab your partner's ankles, and adjust your torso.

19. SPOONING SEX

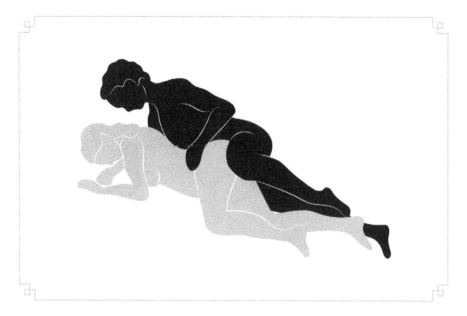

Complexity 🔥 🔥 🔥 🔥 🔥

You may already know this technique for cuddling. The two partners are lying down on their side, the butt of the woman in contact with his genitals. They look like two spoons positioned side by side, and this explains the name. To adjust this position for tantric sex, the lady lies on one side with the knees a bit bent, while the male partner lies on her upper side coming from the back. For the penetration, her legs should open a bit more to allow him to access, and then you can adjust the position once you are connected, making yourselves comfortable. Since the giver partner is coming from the back, this technique is ideal for stimulating her G-Spot. You can try this position also for anal sex.

Hint: Make use of your free arms to cuddling each other. With this position, the giver can kiss his partner's neck and ear if she likes it.

20. Serpent's Embrace

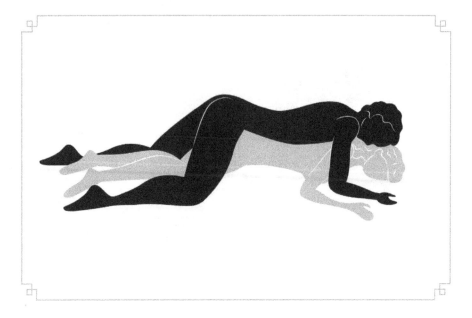

Complexity

This position reminds the spooning one, but instead of being on the side, the woman lies face-down, with a pillow under her hips to raise them a bit. Her forearms are planted on the ground to support her upper body and prop it up slightly. The male partner lies face-down on top of the lady, penetrating her from the back.

Hint: After some time in this position, I suggest the lady moving her legs over the man's shoulders. With this variation, the penetrating part can reach the G-Spot easily and experience some jolts of great pleasure.

21. ROW HIS BOAT

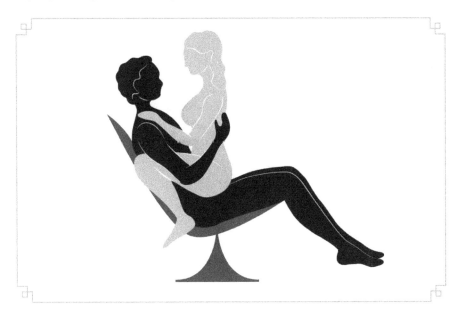

Complexity 🔥🔥🔥🔥🔥

For this position, the male part sits on a chair or sofa with the legs slightly spread. The lady sits on him, straddling his lap and facing him. Her legs are bent and open, passing under his arms, and the feet should lend against the seat of the chair. In this technique, the woman rides him, and she is in charge of the sexual activity. You can use your free arms for cuddling a little; your faces are also pretty close to each other so that you can exchange sweet kisses on the lips. During the waiving, the girl should try with different paces. Another suggestion is to make wide circular movements when thrusting.

Hint: The secret for this position is, for the man, to don't sit straight but to lean back a little. Try this position on a reclining chair to feel more comfortable.

22. WOW-HIM POWWOW

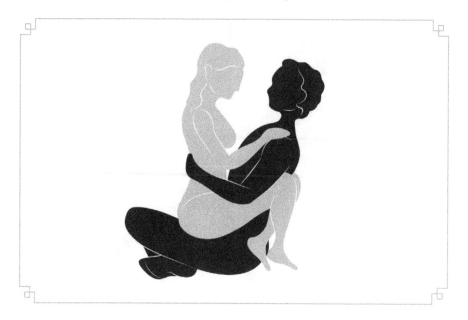

Complexity 🔥🔥🔥🔥🔥

This position is a slight variation of the Yan Yum. First, the man sits down with crossed legs while the lady sits on his lap facing him, leading his penis inside her vagina when sitting. Later, she wraps her legs around his torso while he leans backward a little. Then, holding each other's backs tightly, the couple should start to wave back and forth together, increasing the speed while getting used to the movement.

Hint: Change the way you move to try different levels of intimacy. You can speed up or slow down, get deep, or having shallow penetrations. Try different combinations find the combo that you like most.

23. Sofa Spread-Eagle

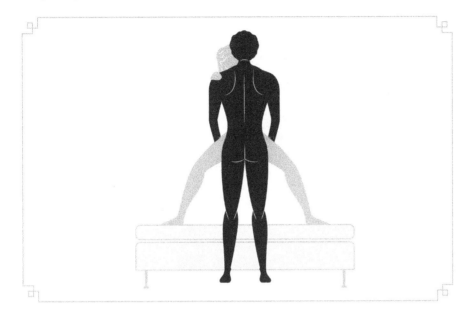

Complexity 🖤 🖤 🖤 🖤 🖤

The lady stands on the edge of a sofa or bed, with her legs spread wide. The man approaches her from the front, standing on the floor. The girl should adjust the height of her stance, extending the legs and bending her knees, while the man should stand straight.

Hint: The pelvises should be at the same level. If she is in a too high position, the man can help by adding some extra height under his feet.

24. HOT SEAT

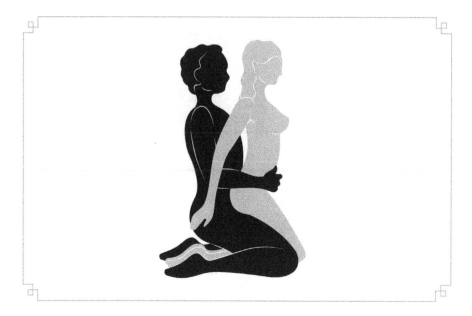

Complexity

The Hot Seat reminds the Yab Yun with the couple facing in the same direction instead of staring at each other. The male part kneels behind the girl, but he has to lean slightly backward. The lady kneels in front of him with the legs between his legs. Her back is touching his front part, and the bodies are squeezed together tightly. The giver's arms can go around her waist, while her hands can grab his forearms or hips. Once connected, try different depths, pressure, and speed.

Hint: When the giver is coming from the back, it's easier for the male member to touch the female G-Spot. The girl should try to swivel her hips in circular motions to stimulate this magic area even better.

25. GET DOWN ON IT

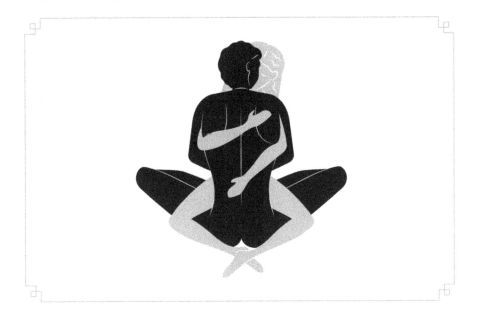

Complexity 🔥 🔥 🔥 🔥 🔥

This position is basically like the Yan Yum with some extra techniques helping with the synchronization between you and your partner. The man sits in the easy pose (with his legs crossed), and the woman sits on him, facing him and wrapping her legs around his waist. They should embrace each other and alternate their breaths, so when one inhales, the other exhales and vice versa. As the lady breathes in, rock your pelvis back and tighten the vaginal muscles. When she exhales, tilt the pelvis forward and release. The two parts should mirror each other.

Hint: Yoga fanatics would probably love this position since it helps with the perfect synchronization between the two lovers. For better intimacy, close your eyes and stay focus on your partner's breath. Don't rush to the waving; try to manage the mirroring of the breath first, and once you get used to it, you can apply the movements. The secret of this technique is to take it slow and relax.

~ CHAPTER 9 ~
Orgasm

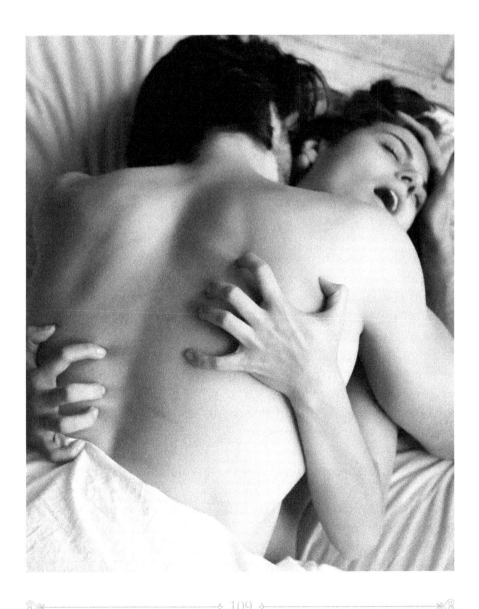

As most people probably already know, an orgasm is a sexual climax. The word orgasm is based on a Greek term meaning "to swell." In Tantra, orgasm is seen as a spiritual experience. But in following the Tantric tradition of slow lovemaking, the goal is generally to prolong orgasm as long as possible.

Many people are getting into Tantra in the last decade to add some fun into their relationship or overcome some issues when making love. Either way, Tantra approaches the experience of sex in a way that makes it supreme and unique. Unfortunately, the ordinary life in the society where we live is causing stress and disorder in our system, and these problems may manifest during sex, blocking us from the satisfaction that we deserve.

Tantric orgasm is about rejecting judgment and breathing into the moment. It's all about focusing the enrgies to finally realise them.

9.1 ORGASM FOR HER

Tantra does not simply provide a way to enhance the sexual experience; it even addresses women's challenges when taking part in sexual relations. For example, it is a common belief in the Tantric philosophy that the most crucial sex organ for a woman is her mind. This organ is where negative thoughts and feelings are born, sometimes negatively affecting sexual desire or the ease of mind necessary to achieve pleasure. Therefore, understanding these feelings and what caused them can help the woman find self-confidence in sex and make her more involved in sexual relations.

We should also consider a common misconception that sees the vagina as a separated part of the female's anatomy. Still, it's much more complex than that. The vagina is not a passive organ but a complex anatomic structure with an active role in sexual arousal and intercourse. The dynamic interactions between the clitoris, urethra and antcrior vaginal are part of the same complex clitourethrovaginal (CUV) system. This complex structure covers a large multifaceted morphofunctional area that, when properly stimulated, could bring to the big O. Here a few techniques that will help a woman in achieving a fantastic orgasm.

Explosive orgasm and implosive orgasm

A woman's orgasmic experience involves multiple erogenous zones in a hard-to-describe mix of sensations. Therefore, it is difficult to classify the various types of orgasms in their various facets. Still, we can use two macro-categories:

- **Explosive orgasm:** It can be represented by a powerful emanation of energy outside the woman's body.
- **Implosive orgasm:** Aims to a greater form of satisfaction.

The **explosive orgasm** involves the genital area and the lower chakras (the Base Chakra - the first - and the Sacral chakra - the second). These orgasms frequently leave a sense of fatigue and disappointment since it does not lead to the total satisfaction of mind and body. Clitoral orgasm is of this kind.

The **implosive orgasm** is an experience in which the energy doesn't scatter outside but collapses inwards, involving the upper chakras. It can include the entire body, just as the psychological and passionate circles of the lady, conveying a general sense of satisfaction and contentment. These types of orgasms are both physical and mental. The vaginal orgasm and the cervical-uterine orgasm are of this sort.

Clitoral Stimulation

Believe it or not, but there are ways for a woman to reach orgasm without passing through the penetration phase. In fact, according to a 2017 study, only about 18 percent of women achieve orgasm through penetration. Clitoral stimulation is beneficial when it comes to orgasming during sex. I mentioned before how the clitoris is such a receptive spot that it is even more sensitive than the men's penis. Of course, sex, in itself, is a critical stimulating demonstration; anyway, the clitoris is the pearl that gives the vast majority of the sexual joy that a woman experiences. For this reason, it is essential to focus on this area as much as possible before and during sex. It is important to be as gentle as possible when stimulating this area due to its incredible sensitivity.

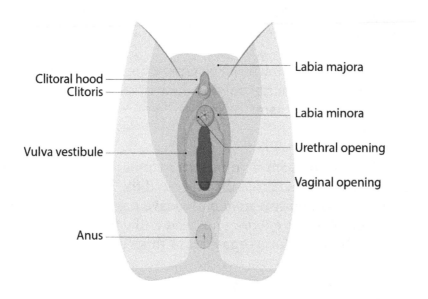

G-Spot

The exercises of Tantra show that there is a holy spot inside a woman's vagina called G-Spot, which is extremely sensitive. If stimulated correctly, this area can convey high peaks of pleasure for a woman. The "G" of the G-spot comes from Gräfenberg, a German physician and scientist who invented an intra-uterine device for his studies about female orgasm. His experiments revealed that there is a particular area inside the female reproductive system that produces intense stimulus. This spot can be easily found when performing the "come here" motion with the middle finger inside the vagina.

However, recent studies clarify that the G-Spot isn't a separated area of women's anatomy, but it's part of the clitoral network. So, stimulating the G-Spot is like stimulating the clitoris from the inside. Turns out, the little nub coming out where the inner labia meet is only the tip of the clitoris. Even if this magic area can be spotted with the "come here" motion of your finger, consider that this region varies from woman to woman, so there are cases where it's challenging to find the correct position. Anyway, it's worth it for a woman to explore her body and to locate her G-spot because once discovered, sex will move to much higher levels.

Cervical-uterine Orgasm

The cervical-uterine orgasm is much less famous than the clitoral and G-spot ones because it's not as common as the previous two, and it's not straightforward to recognize it. The cervix is a cylinder-shaped neck of tissue that connects the vagina and uterus. So to get to the cervix, it's going to involve deep penetration.

The area surrounded by the cervix presents many nerves distributed throughout the entire pelvis, so pressing this area or rubbing against it may bring the woman to an intense sense of pleasure.

Aiming for a cervical orgasm is not a simple thing; as said, the cervix is in a pretty deep position, then you may require a relatively long member to reach it. Also, each vagina has a different design, so you may need a particular angle or curve to get to the right spot.

If you want to try this experience, it may be an exciting journey to try also with your partner, especially if you are keen to attempt new experiments in bed. Most of the positions coming from behind are ideal for exploring the cervix zone; also, you may consider using a toy to amplify your research.

9.2 Orgasm for him

It is customary to believe that, for men, the orgasm manifests through ejaculation. Achieving this status is indeed the result of great pleasure. Still, the feeling of ecstasy usually lasts just a few moments before it gradually disappears and what follows is the lowest condition of sexual excitement for a man. After the peak, the man usually loses his interest, and he needs to wait some time before reactivating his sexual desire. For this reason, ejaculation is usually the end of lovemaking, which, on some occasions, may leave the woman not fully satisfied.

If you are a man, I know what you may be thinking: "How can I last longer? How can I limit my pleasure and delay my final orgasm?" Before answering it, I want to raise something that most people usually forget. Ejaculation and orgasm are two different things. Indeed you can have an orgasm that manifests through ejaculation, but they don't have necessarily come together.

In the end, orgasm is something happening in your mind. It's the feeling of immense pleasure coming from the stimulus applied to your body. When you perceive many peaks in a short period, you are getting a multiorgasm, and the ecstasy coming from it is a much more incredible feeling than whatever you'll ever sense when ejaculating.

Multiorgasm and long sexual intercourse are directly related. If you have a long and intense sensual activity, you'll get more chances to reach the multiorgasm. To achieve both results, you need to take control of your body and master your sperma release; in doing so, you'll decide the duration of your lovemaking. Don't worry. Over thousands of years, the participants in tantric sex have mastered different methods to control their ejaculation, and this section is about sharing some of those secrets.

How to last longer

The first thing to last longer is to don't ejaculate early. Ok, this is too obvious. How do you actually do that? It's pretty simple, and it's also the most difficult thing to do: don't think about ejaculating. When you are making love, you don't have to think about the grand finale; actually, you don't have to think about anything at all! In tantra is all about feeling the moment. So, clear your mind and enjoy all the pleasure coming from the experience. For this reason, relaxation is such an essential key in tantra. When you relax, your thoughts are silent, and your mind is free to enjoy any sensations coming through your body. I know. It's not very simple to don't think about ejaculating but starting with the idea to reject it is the first step for you to delay it as far as you can.

All the tantric secrets discussed until now have the purpose of reaching awareness and getting better control of your body. Therefore, all the techniques to practice tantra can help you to achieve long-sex endurance. Yoga, meditation, and pranayamas are all fundamental parts if you want to reach ejaculation-mastery. But, from all, the essential one is breath control. In tantra, you use your breath to connect with your partner. How you breathe also decides the rhythm of your lovemaking, and in tantric sex, you want to go slow. So, whenever you feel close to the peak, slow down your breath even more: try with five seconds breathing in and five seconds breathing out. If you feel comfortable, you can even try to hold your breath for a couple of seconds occasionally.

To master the control of your peak, you can also train specifically the part of your body that causes the ejaculation. I am talking about the PC muscle (or pubococcygeus muscle), situated between the pubic bone and the tail bone, forming the floor of your pelvic cavity. This muscle contracts during ejaculation and controls the urine activity too.

Now that you are aware of the existence of the PC muscle, you need to understand how to take control of it. The method is the same that you apply when you are holding your urine. To make it in practice, you can try to stop the flow while you are peeing. Next time you have to urinate, give it a try: stop the flow and then release it, stop it again and then release it, and so on. This will make you aware of the muscle that you need to train. Now that you know about this muscle, you don't have to necessary pee to improve its strength. Just contract it regularly during your everyday life, like sitting at a desk or waiting for the bus. This practice is called **Kegel exercise**, also known as **pelvic-floor exercise.**

Applying this training with regularity is a very healthy habit, not only for taking control of the ejaculation. But you need to be patient and constant with this activity because it takes about three months to see the results. Still, I promise it will be worth it! Reinforcing the pelvic floor muscle is beneficial for both women and men because it helps prevent continence and pre-ejaculation issues. Women can apply the Kegel exercise too, but I will talk about this later.

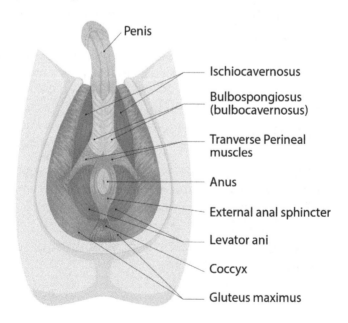

Pompoir

There is an exciting female-centered technique in tantra where the man is slowly stimulated by the contraction of the vagina. Pompoir is a sexual technique where the woman is entirely in charge of the activity while the man is totally passive; still, he gets the best fun. This technique is also known as *kabzah*, and is also referred to as *Singapore Kiss*. The woman typically goes on the top, and she grabs and holds the partner's member contracting her vaginal muscles. The stimulation comes through muscle contraction alone, and no other actions are required, like rocking or thrusting. So, it requires much vaginal strength and contraction skills; but once the woman acquires these abilities, she will be able to provide her man one of the best sensations in his life. Training your body to apply this technique requires time and constant practice, and you need to wait from four to six months to perform it correctly. You can even use some tools to accelerate your training, like Yoni eggs or Ben wa balls, but they are in no way necessary. In the next section, I'll give you some exercises to learn how to perform pompoir for your man.

For women: practicing Pompoir

Pompoir is an action caused through the vaginal muscles to stimulate the man's member when making love with your partner. This act is meant to give pleasure to the male partner, but it's also beneficial for the woman since it gives her more empowerment during tantric sex. Having the female partner practicing with pompoir improves the sexual experience for both the subjects. Unfortunately, this practice is mainly known in Far Eastern cultures, and it arrived in the Western world just recently, especially when you come to known the tantric world.

Pompoir is not an easy skill because it's happening internally. But there are four main motions to focus on when practicing it: squeeze, contract, push and pull. But before describing these actions, let's start with the basics. I mentioned before the Kegel exercise, and I gave some instructions for the men to perform it. Now, it's time to provide some guidance for the women.

Some women may already hear about the Kegel exercises since many doctors recommend it during and after pregnancy to help prevent urinary leaking. To apply this training, you can place your finger inside your vagina and try to squeeze it with the muscles in your pelvic. Another way to practicing is to try to stop your urine mid-flow, thigh and hold for few seconds and then relax. But the last one is just a suggestion to figure out the feeling and the muscles you need to train for the pompoir. Holding your urine regularly, even for few seconds, is not a good practice for a healthy reason, so once you realized the action you need to replicate, practice with it without putting your health on the line. Once you have figured out how to squeeze your pelvic muscle, you can take any possible occasion to compress and release during your daily routine.

Once you get better with squeezing through Kegel exercises, you can try the next step: pull and push. For these actions, you need to imagine that your vagina is sucking something and than pulling it out. The movements are the same as the Kegel exercise, but you need some practice before getting it right. My suggestion is to try to understand these actions involving your partner. Next time you are busy in lovemaking, explain to your partner what you want to perform and ask him to thrust slowly. Then, with your vagina muscles, do the opposite of what he is doing: when he moves in, you push out, like if you are trying to reject him out; when he pulls out, you squeeze as you want to suck him in. This is a good training to understand how to perform it, and having your partner involved will definitely add some fun! Once you get familiar with the movements, you can practice them yourself like you are doing with the previous exercise. To perform it alone, you'll better do it on the toilet; sitting on something hollow will help you put effort into the correct muscles while the rest of the body is relaxing.

Once you acquire some skills with the pull-push, you may want to try the "twisting." As the name suggests, imagine holding a pen between the thumb and the pointer finger, and you move it from one side to the other, twisting the pen. You have to replicate the same movements with your pelvic muscles when your partner is inside you. With this type of action, not only will your man be swallowed by a wave of pleasure, but you too will enjoy his member moving around your vaginal tissue.

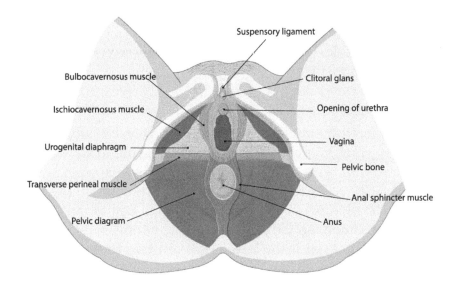

9.3 MULTIPLE ORGASMS AND LONG ORGASM

Orgasm is the final goal when having sex, and people want this experience to be excellent and unique. If having an orgasm generates the most incredible feeling of pleasure and satisfaction, having more than one in a short period can only make the experience even better. Take in mind, however, that the multiorgasm is not the final goal for tantric sex. On the contrary, people who practice Tantra aim to get one single orgasm that can last for a long time. Some veterans in tantric sex may claim to experience orgasms that may have last even half an hour.

Multiorgasm and tantric orgasm are two different experiences because however long an orgasm lasts, it's still just one orgasm.

Multiple orgasms, instead, require the first orgasm to end before starting a new one later, so there is like a break between them where the subject is relaxing a bit. Typically, the multiorgasm happens through continued or renewed stimulation.

Saying if the multiorgasm experience is worst or better than a long-period orgasm is entirely subjective. Some people may prefer one or the other depending on their idea of great pleasure. Either way, both the experiences are worth trying, and tantric sex can help make them happen. Following some guidelines to help you with them.

Keep your cool

This may sound unusual, yet the best way by which you can defer your intercourse is by keeping your cool. On the off chance that you feel that your peak is snappy moving closer, you have to calm down, limiting your breathing and pushing developments. Remember that one key to tantric sex is communication, so let your accomplice know why you are slowing down, even if the best is for you two to agree on the same goals before starting the intercourse.

Go gradually

When you start participating in tantric sex with your accomplice, guarantee that you are taking things progressively. The more slow the sex is, the more outstanding your peak would be, an immediate consequence of all the turn of events.

Calm yourself, obstruct your breathing, and handle your pelvic muscles.

When you feel that your peak is subsiding, relax a bit and calm down your breath; after a short time, you can eventually proceed with your pushing development. Keep repeating this methodology for whatever time that you can hold off. Develop your energy and keep going. This advancement will make your peak last more, and it will be even more noteworthy. When you feel that you are close to peak, endeavor and grasp your pubic muscles while still going on. It will not simply hold you back from releasing; it will also allow you to encounter the joy of a peak and not lose your erection, which means that you will be able to prop up extensively in the wake of experiencing an orgasm. After some practice, you will have the alternative to hold off for quite a while longer and participate in sexual relations for a significant long time together.

Conclusion

When you learn about tantric sex, you realize how the perception built around the act of love is a matter of mindset. Some people feel guilty when talking about sex and prefer to keep all their naughty experiences locked away. Others may talk about sex shamelessly and feel proud of their achievements and performances. Sex in modern life is a topic full of contradictions and challenges. It's described as one of the most beautiful experiences in life, but at the same time, it is considered a perverted and sinful act.

Considering these contradictions, it's pretty clear why some couples feel reluctant to talk about sex, sometimes even between each other. Whatever you are facing troubles in your relationship or looking for new tips and emotions to bring into your sexual activity, finding the right person and moment to ask for advice can be challenging.

This is where Tantra can come as an answer for some couples facing this dilemma. Tantra is a journey that opens our minds and can help us to live with harmony and accept divinity in our lives. It teaches how to find balance, accept pleasure and feelings as they come, and make use of them to contemplate the beauty of the material and spiritual world. Although most people associate Tantra only with sex, it's a much deeper discipline. Following, I want to summarize some of the teachings I learned along my journey, hoping that they can come in handy for you while finding your own path.

It's not only about sex

Associate tantra automatically to sex is a misconception. Tantra is not about prolonged and uncontrolled sexual intercourse, as assumed by many. Sex is a primary instinct instilled in human nature to ensure the species survive. Tantra has a much deeper meaning; it does make use of sexual energy in a constructive way. Through Tantra, we want to explore our limitations and overcome them.

For this reason, Tantra is neither a religion nor a science but a spiritual journey. It's an instrument that allows the individual to deeper understand themselves and improve through the development of mind and body. The objective of Tantra is to have the option to work with your accomplice together to accomplish an absolute pleasure and cause the other individual to feel better. In any case, you don't need orgasm as the objective. Instead, you should cooperate to make yourself both upbeat and fulfilled.

It's about knowing your body

Like yoga, tantra is all about physical and spiritual awareness. When you walk the path of tantra, you take more consciousness about your body and your areas of pleasure. There is nothing to be ashamed about; you need to consider yourself as a divinity, and your body is the temple that brings you to heaven. Remember that the word "tantra" means "to wave" because everything is connected, as your body is connected to your internal energy that flows in powerful waves. Knowing yourself is the first step to get in contact with your spirit and the entire Universe.

It's about knowing your partner

In most cases, when a couple approaches Tantra is to add some fun into their relationship. Indeed, Tantra may sound exciting and inspiring, but it's also a discipline that requires seriousness and devotion. When you apply tantric teachings with your partner, you start a spiritual journey together, which can bring the two of you to a profound bond. Using Tantra in a relationship means to be physically aware and spiritually present for each other. You approve to exchange your energies with one another, keeping this connection even after the orgasm. Staring this journey together will allow you to understand each other better. This is not only about discovering the erogenous zones of your partner's body but exploring their soul.

You Might not Get it Right the First Time

Most people approach Tantra to have better and longer sex, and they expect to get results in short times. But there are no such things as short-cuts in life, and Tantra is no exception. So, whatever is the reason that brings you close to this philosophy, you will have to try multiple times before seeing any results. You may search for the best sex in your life, or maybe you are just willing to bring some fun into your relationship, but if you don't practice, you'll never get whatever you want to achieve. It's a sort of training that requires persistence, and you should consistently put aside the time you go through with your partner. So, don't get frustrated if you won't see any changes the first time you are doing tantric sex. Don't give up at the beginning, and you'll get there one step per time.

Take it slow and enjoy the trip

We are so busy with everyday life that we don't have time to relax and enjoy the beauty in the world. With sex, the problem is similar. We rush so much to reach the orgasm, and in the end, we'll end up with bitter and incomplete satisfaction. Tantra teaches the opposite. To take things slow, to enjoy the moment, and to relax instead of rushing. This teaching is applied for Tantra in sex as in life. Too often, we live in expectations, and we are too busy aiming the target that we are blind to everything else. It's good to set up goals because they lead us to what we want, and they give us the time to organize. Even for tantric sex, it's a good practice to have it planned with your partner to have everything ready in time. But starting with a goal in mind doesn't necessarily mean ignoring whatever is not on your path. Sometimes it's nice to step back and enjoy the journey.

I am aware that Tantra is a very profound discipline and this book scratches only the surface of the topic. My purpose was to give you some basic knowledge about this fascinating culture without neglecting the fun that comes with it. I did my best to cover both theory and practice to provide you with a general understanding and getting you in touch with the basics. Now it's up to you to decide to go deep with this path and apply it regularly in your everyday life or use the knowledge provided for occasional fun. Either way, I hope this book will guide you along your journey and contribute to improving your life.

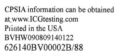
CPSIA information can be obtained
at www.ICGtesting.com
Printed in the USA
BVHW090809140122
626140BV00002B/88